Praise for *Tales from the Crib*

"In these bite-sized, hilariou[...]s the
underachiever in all of us. Any[...]ff in the
same yoga pants she slept in w[...]nd feel a
w[...]
—Amy Wilson, author of *When Did I Get Like This?*

"A fun romp through the messy realities of being a mom. DeeDee Filiatreault
writes with humor, and from the heart . . ."
—Christie Mellor, author of *The Three-Martini Playdate*
and *Fun Without Dick and Jane*

"By page 10, I was nodding in agreement. By page 110, I was convinced
DeeDee and I were leading parallel lives. By the end, I wanted her to
move next door—with or without her children. *Tales from the Crib* will
make you smile and laugh, especially if your kids are finally asleep in their
beds—or anywhere, really."
—Leanne Shirtliffe, author of *Don't Lick the Minivan* and *Mommyfesto*

"DeeDee's stories are laugh-out-loud funny and worth embarrassing yourself
over—whether on the train, the bus, the subway, or even in your own bathroom.
Or someone else's bathroom. DeeDee is our generation's Erma Bombeck!"
—Todd Ellison, Broadway music supervisor of
An American in Paris, *Spamalot*, and *42nd Street*

"DeeDee Filiatreault has been there, done that, and kept a sense of humor
throughout the journey of motherhood. She hands out 'honorable mention'
ribbons to all of the parents and confirms there is no 'right way' to parent—just
our way."
—Val Curtis, editor-in-chief of BonBon Break Media, LLC

"DeeDee has a rare gift—she can make you laugh about things you didn't know
were funny until she pointed them out, and she can make a quasi-serious point
at the same time. These essays are terrific."
—Barton Swaim, author of *The Speechwriter: A Brief Education in Politics*

"DeeDee Filiatrealt is a modern-day Erma Bombeck. In her transparent, witty,
and extremely well-written debut release, *Tales from the Crib*, DeeDee strips
away the pretenses of parenthood, modeling the medicinal power of laughter
and how to celebrate the joy in every jelly stain. Her writing is a gift."
—Tara McClary Reeves, author of *Point Me to Jesus*

TALES FROM THE CRIB

TALES FROM THE CRIB

ADVENTURES OF AN OVER-SHARING,
STRESSED-OUT, MODERN-DAY MOM

DEEDEE FILIATREAULT

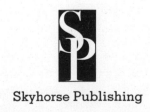

Skyhorse Publishing

Memoirs, by definition, are written depictions of events in people's lives. They are memories. All the events in this story are as accurate and truthful as possible. Many names and places have been changed to protect the privacy of others. Mistakes, if any, are caused solely by the passage of time.

Skyhorse Publishing books may be purchased in bulk at special discounts for sales promotion, corporate gifts, fund-raising, or educational purposes. Special editions can also be created to specifications. For details, contact the Special Sales Department, Skyhorse Publishing, 307 West 36th Street, 11th Floor, New York, NY 10018or info@skyhorsepublishing.com.

Skyhorse® and Skyhorse Publishing® are registered trademarks of Skyhorse Publishing, Inc.®, a Delaware corporation.

Visit our website at www.skyhorsepublishing.com.

10 9 8 7 6 5 4 3 2 1

Library of Congress Cataloging-in-Publication Data is available on file.

Cover design by Jenny Zemanek
Cover photo credit iStock

Print ISBN: 978-1-63450-684-7
Ebook ISBN: 978-1-63450-685-4

Printed in the United States of America

For Bill, Willis, and Lucy
You're what this book (and my life) are all about . . . or whatever.

"When you slip on a banana peel, people laugh at you. But when you tell people you slipped on a banana peel, it's your laugh."

—Nora Ephron

"We writers are not nouns. We are mere adjectives, serving the great Noun of truth."

—C. S. Lewis

CONTENTS

INTRODUCTION

Dear friend,

You know it, and I know it: you will probably end up reading this book on the toilet.

But please, rest assured—I am 100 percent okay with that.

Because let's face it, if you're reading this, chances are good that: a) you have kids, and b) you've been known to seek sanctuary in the bathroom. (Never mind the child's heavy breathing through the crack in the door, the pounding, the hollering, or the notes slid underneath. Bathroom-hiding has never been a foolproof plan, but it's all we've got.)

This book is perfect for those moments of "quiet."

You hold in your hands a compendium of columns and blogs I've written over the past decade or so—all of them about the foibles of our family life and all of which should make you feel a whole lot better about yourself as a parent. You can churn through one in five minutes or less and leave the water closet feeling refreshed, encouraged, and perhaps a bit superior.

So please, don't feel any shame if this becomes your toilet book. I'm just happy you're reading it.

Actually, some of the most formative reading of my life has happened in the bathroom.

Growing up in North Carolina, a basket always sat nestled next to our harvest gold family toilet, filled with a decade's worth of dusty back issues of *Guideposts* and *Reader's Digest* and sometimes (when we were especially *au courant*) a relatively recent *Newsweek*. Looking back now, I realize these were probably the filthiest, germiest magazines of all time and should never have been handled without latex gloves and a charcoal-filtered breathing mask.

But handle them I did. In five-minute snatches throughout my adolescence, *Guideposts* shaped my thoughts on God with its real-life accounts of miracles, answered prayers, and angels in disguise. *Reader's Digest* told me my first jokes—most of them riddled with puns and corn—but that didn't keep me from running to recite them to my dad when I was all done in there. (*Newsweek* would have infused me with global understanding on topics like Beirut and Imelda Marcos if I'd read those parts, but I mostly stuck to the movie reviews.)

All that bathroom reading made me who I am today. Perhaps this book can do the same for you. (Or not. But it *is* something to do in there.) I don't have any cool angel stories, but I have more than my fair share about mammograms, soccer practice, and trying to wedge myself into skinny jeans. I'm guessing you do, too, so *boom*. Instant friends, ready to dish.

My first *Tales from the Crib* column appeared in our local Connecticut weekly in 2007. I wrote—with great sappiness—about our oldest child starting preschool with his tiny dinosaur backpack. (At best, you could pack a box of sixty-four Crayolas in that thing, maybe a snack. Today, he totes his own middle-school body weight on his back.)

I'd reached that slightly less immersive place in early motherhood where I could breathe a little easier, think a little clearer, and write a little now and then—about *them*, of course. I'd always used writing as a tool for remaining a sane, high-functioning adult and making a living. Other than counted cross-stitch, it's the most impressive skill I have.

So I started writing what I knew around our "crib," always striving for the sweet spot between protecting my children's feelings and putting it all out there. I wrestled the kooky stuff of family life onto the page and tried to make sense out of it—partly for my own sanity, partly for the laugh.

But when you try to be as real as you can, you're just begging for someone to call you a bad mother—like that kind lady who emailed me to say, "You shouldn't have children, let alone a dog." (I may cross-stitch that on a pillow someday.)

The thing is, on my less than optimum parenting days, I tend to agree with her. Some days, when I want to go into the Witness Protection Program just for a couple nights, when I (ahem) *do not handle things well*, I wonder how I could possibly be *worse* at this job.

But if we're honest, all of us who devote eighteen-plus years of our lives to this parenting business are bound to have those doom-and-gloom thoughts from time to time. Because none of us could ever be fully equipped for the grinding minutia of this mammoth task. We're just not.

Yet when the grocery cart is overflowing with a writhing toddler, when the sippy cup of milk drenches the seat cushions, when the tween is glowering into her breakfast cereal, we're supposed to be able to magically call upon the highlighted sections of that stack of parenting books on the bedside table and respond with loving, lightning-fast, Dr. Spock–like wisdom.

Sometimes—praises be!—we do, and all who bear witness marvel at our patience and wisdom.

But sometimes, we just don't parent to perfection. Sometimes we epically fail, and those are the moments when, I think, we have to laugh.

Oh sure, pray for help and forgiveness first. And definitely go back and highlight those books again, this time in hot pink to make sure it takes.

But somewhere in there—preferably before, after, and in-between—you have to laugh.

That's what I've tried to do with what I write—to find the laugh. I want you to feel like I'm a friend you can crack up with while seated at my sticky dining table, the one covered with the detritus of last week's unexamined Friday Folders and dotted with imitation maple syrup from last night's pancake supper.

So just push aside those piles of school papers, forgotten dental bills, and artwork I can't bear to throw away, and pull up a chair.

When you do, I hope you'll feel less alone. I hope you'll find a friend in these pages who won't judge you for your Lunchables if you won't judge her for her dust rabbits (we're way past bunnies). I hope you'll even glimpse a Friend who knows all our failings and still—by some miracle—manages to work through us for good. His table is where real meaning is found. (It also happens to be made of solid gold without a single crumb anywhere. But don't let that put you off. He can't help being perfect, and He gets that we're not.)

So thank you again for reading this. I know you don't have much time, and you could just as easily flip through a J.Crew catalog during your five-minute escape.

But I promise you this—I will make you feel way better about yourself than that skinny girl with her messy bun and pencil skirt.

So read on, my friend. May your next five minutes be five luxurious, laughter-filled minutes well spent—or your money back.

Actually, forget that part. It's too late for that. But still, I really hope you like the book.

Your friend,
DeeDee

PART I

TROPHIES FOR
SHOWING UP

Hi. I'm an Honorable Mention. Nice to meet you. I'm guessing you're one, too.

Honorable Mention is the ribbon I was forever coming home with (usually in some non-winning, non-primary color like chartreuse) every field day of my youth. After staggering across the finish line dead last in a potato sack or tied to some poor sap who was quick to regret her choice of a partner, I'd stuff my Honorable Mention in the nearest, deepest pocket and cast an envious glance at everyone else's sparkly blue ones.

What does *Honorable Mention* even mean? That it's an honor just to be mentioned in the same breath as other faster, sleeker, more-likely-to-succeed types? That I should be honored to have this loser ribbon instead of jack squat (which is what I deserve but everyone's too kind to say so)?

I guess it just means there was at least some shred of honor in showing up and giving it the old middle-school try. (Kids on the losing team today get three-foot-tall trophies just for showing up. The price of coddling has really skyrocketed.)

Thirty years later, I've hung up my potato sack.

My grown-up life is now spent on the *parenting* fields—coaching, cheering, patching up, praying like Tim Tebow, taking the occasional knee. I work crazy hours. I eat, sleep, and breathe it.

But the scoreboard doesn't lie. I'm still kicking a solid Honorable Mention. I'm still not quite up to the loftiest blue-ribbon standards.

My guess is they reserve the blue ones for moms who whip up Halloween costumes with something other than a credit card, laminate chore charts for the fridge, and prep all the crafts for class parties. (Or maybe those are the moms who are weird clean freaks or are always half an hour late. We've all got our issues.)

But I'll go out on a limb here and say this—we are *all* Honorable Mentions.

Oh sure, we're all capable of scoring a solid blue ribbon every now and then. (God likes to give us a taste of winning to keep us thinking we can actually *do* this.) But consistently, day in and day out, most of us remain squarely average, ordinary, run-of-the-mill Mothers of the Chartreuse Ribbon.

It's just that hard to be awesome at this all the time.

On any given Sunday, we could rock it or we could get creamed. We could sway along to "We are the Champions" or we could get pelted with tomatoes.

Such is the reality of parenting. Not everything in family life is worthy of the highlight reel. Not everything you try is a touchdown pass. The essays in this section are all about being good enough, even if we're never quite as good as it gets.

But mom (and dad, too), if you are holding this book in your hands, I already know this about you. You are someone who's leaving it all on the field—your days, nights, energy, dignity, brains, tears, prayers, down time, bank account, girlish figure, solid nine at night, dreams of international travel, and clean carpets—your whole heart.

What you're doing is a thing of honor.

I just thought I'd mention it.

In Celebration of Supermom
May 2010

Motherhood, they say, is a Herculean task.

And by Herculean, they're referring to a dude who slayed lions *and* a hydra with nine heads *and* still managed to clean the biggest, smelliest stables in the land in a single day. (At least that's what Wikipedia says.)

So if we moms are anything like that guy, I'd say we're nothing short of superheroes.

(Watch me as I stretch these superhero parallels thinner than George Clooney's Batman tights.)

Allow me to introduce to you: Supermom.

Supermom works incognito, often under cover of darkness, in a world where her good deeds go largely unrecognized. As though hidden behind a nerdy pair of Clark Kent specs, she does all the hard stuff that ultimately changes the world—but without fanfare or headlines.

Supermom is maniacally protective of the citizens of her personal Gotham. She will all but turn green and bust through the sleeves of her favorite Loft sweater set if anybody messes with her kid.

Supermom can suppress the gag reflex in the face of even the most stomach-churning calamities. (I know one hard-core mom who—while trapped in the bleachers at a crowded basketball game—literally opened the buttons of her shirt to give her sick kid a place to throw up. I'd like to see Iron Man do *that*.)

Supermom laughs in the face of danger as she is armed to the teeth with high-tech weaponry, from glue guns to OxiClean.

Supermom's biceps are taut from curling an infant carrier, while her ample backside reflects her commitment to making cupcakes for every notable occasion in her children's lives.

Supermom is capable of reading minds and tracking childhood mischief from the eyes placed strategically in the back of her head. (That stuff's no joke.)

Supermom can contort herself into any elastic position to rescue a dropped pacifier from the backseat floorboard or swat at bickering, back-talking children.

Supermom is a complicated, tormented soul, devoted to doing good, but longing a thousand times a day for a life in which not so much is required of her. She carries on anyway, knowing it is her reason for being.

Supermom *cannot* bend spoons with her mind, leap tall buildings in a single bound, or (let's face it) wear a catsuit anymore. But that's a pretty short list.

So today I raise my cape to all the Supermoms out there committed to truth, justice, and the American way. Never forget you're making the world a better place—one irksome, exasperating, lovable kid at a time.

Life According to Lands´ End (and Other Pretty Lies)

February 2014

Fortnightly, it comes—the Lands' End catalog.

Its pages set the tone for a crisply pressed life of reasonable fashionableness. Nothing too flashy. Nothing too Anthropologie-hipster. Nothing too J.Crew-prepster.

Flipping through the cable-knit pages, I ponder the life of a Lands' Ender, all easy-breezy curls and matching sweater sets. And I shrug to myself, "I could do this, *right*?"

Get a grip, you deludenoid. Not even close.

Let's just feast our eyes on what life would look like if I—your garden-variety, middle-aged mom—were a Lands' End model.

The day would dawn on my zillion-count Egyptian cotton sheets, crisp and blindingly white, without blemish or mascara smudge or yellowing from years of wear and drool.

I would emerge from this cottony cloud in an empire-waist lace cami with matching bottoms rather than my husband, Bill's, Adidas hoodie and droopy flannel pants that God never intended to be capri pants but have become so after repeated washings. There would also be much energetic stretching, smiling, and springing.

I would throw on my Trail Sport Mary Janes, a jog bra (whether I needed it or not), and one of my many pairs of cropped yoga performance pants to wick away all that Pilates-induced sweat rather than staggering straight to the shower without the slightest pretense of exercise today.

I would prepare my adoring children's lunch boxes in my casual jacquard tunic, jewel-toned skinny jeans rolled at the cuff, and cork captoe ballet slippers rather than the same boot-cut jeans I've worn all week, a Goodwill turtleneck that was passably cute circa 2004, and my nubuck house slippers with the threadbare wooly insides. (The brand is called Old Friend, if that tells you anything.)

After the bus whisks away my Hilfiger-esque trophy children, I would sip mimosas on a sailboat with other moms equally comfortable in their own wedge heels rather than plopping down to Facebook and a bowl of Frosted Mini-Wheats. I would never even pause to question if my sparkly children had brushed their teeth.

I would have a monogrammed canvas tote at the ready for every foreseeable need rather than one giant mom purse stuffed with deci-mated granola bars, an ice scraper, and not a single pen that writes.

By my side would be the ultimate go-to accessory—the smiling Labrador retriever in yellow rather than the socially awkward terrier with a fixed look of disappointment.

———————

Nobody's striving for a *Vogue* cover here. This is just Lands' End I'm talking about—home of Sperry Topsiders and the skirted tankini. How is it I still can't pull this off?

Maybe because all of it's *fake*.

Garnet Hill's twelve coordinating pillows for one bed? Fake.

Hanna Andersson's sweet little Nordic sprites in tulle and clogs? So cute, but so fake (*and* so perilous for wee ankles).

Whimsical Instagrams of summer afternoons and snow days? Filtered and fake. (Fess up. You're watching mind-numbing amounts of TV just like the rest of us.)

The ether is filled with so much art-directed, airbrushed hoo-ha that we start believing all that lovely "perfection" is real life—if not for us, then probably for everybody else.

It's not. And if it is for you, I'm not sure we can be friends.

Maybe on my best day, I could rock those teal beads and the Welt Pocket Sheath with coordinating dress cardigan. It's good to have goals. But until I have to meet the president, this is how I roll. It's 2:30 in the afternoon, and I am still in these house shoes.

Multihued espadrilles, they're not, but at least I've got Old Friends.

The Metamorphosis
of Mensa Mom

October 2011

I don't mean to brag, but I am the perfect mother.

That's what my seven-year-old, Will just told me—right after I gave him a fistful of salt and vinegar potato chips.

I know what you're thinking: that actually might make me a *crappy* mother.

Maybe you're one of those people who stocks the fridge with bowlfuls of peapods or berries picked straight from the family garden, ready for "anytime snacking."

I wish I were. Sadly, I am one of those people who counts a Sponge Bob–shaped "fruit snack" as actual fruit and calls it a vitamin-packed day. I have a sneaking suspicion that's one of the reasons my children think I'm perfect. Oh, and they're also too little to know any better.

Working from this blissful state of ignorance, my five-year-old, Lucy, has been making me lots of lovey-dovey art lately. She doodles all manner of rainbows, birdies, and families locking their clown-sized hands together, always under the banner I LOVE MY MOMMY.

I am framing them as evidence. They could prove useful one day when the bright shining light of my perfection starts to fade. Because if the rumor holds true, my metamorphosis isn't too far away.

Soon enough, I will fall from my perch of greatness as Mensa Mom (capable of unlocking such mysteries of the universe as "When was God born?"), only to be reduced to the most clueless excuse for an air-sucking life-form ever to walk the Earth.

I'm told the day is coming when my kids will slink down in the backseat rather than be seen with me, when they'll roll their eyes at the very fact that I'm breathing in and out.

I want to weep at the thought of it—and at the memories of my own clueless parents, whose legacy of awkwardness I seem doomed to repeat.

I remember my mother all too well, ever the chipper camp counselor behind the wheel of the morning carpool, trying (and failing) to rouse a car full of sourpuss teenage girls into vibrato sing-alongs of "This is the Day." Picture teenage-me sweating in hot shame, fumbling for an ejector seat button.

Then there was my dad, arriving light-years too early to pick me up from the eighth-grade dance. I can still see that bald head poking out above a sea of sparkly claw bangs, scanning the crowd for his darling daughter. Phil Collins serenaded as I prayed for the cafeteria floor to swallow me (and my enormous shoulder pads) whole.

Nothing short of electroshock therapy will purge the memories of my parents being dumb and embarrassing. It just took a few years of smartening up before I could see they weren't actually all that dumb (but still plenty embarrassing; my dad has a thing for puns and inadvertent gas passing).

At least for this lovely little honeymoon phase, my daughter still waves and presses her face against that germy bus window until she can't see mine anymore.

It's weird, but she loves my face—last night's makeup and all. A five-year-old's mother is truly a noble subject worthy of art, song, and praise.

Mine is a tenuous grip on perfection. I know it won't last. Bubbles burst. Children grow up. Perfect mommies get outgrown.

My day is coming when I'll embarrass the crap out of my children (sometimes on purpose), when I'll be woefully out-of-touch and not know who Selena Gomez is, when I'll "ruin their lives" with lame rules about texting and tank tops.

But I'm counting on it all coming full circle when they grow up and realize they had it right the first time. Heck yeah, I was dumb and embarrassing. But I also gave them a lifetime supply of love, support, *and* fruit snacks.

That makes me as close to a perfect mother as they'll ever get.

Cracking the Teacher Conference Code

November 2014

It's parent-teacher conference season—that hap-hap-happy time of year when we get slapped in the face with all our finest parental failings.

Don't get me wrong—I'm a huge fan of all my kids' teachers. They are smart, lovely people who aren't paid enough for their troubles.

But I will say this about teachers as a whole: whether they're trying to spare our feelings or avoid coming off like total jerks, *they speak in code.*

So today I'm going to be your sassy, straight-talking friend (your own personal Jackée, if you will) and translate "nice teacher" into "plain English" for you.

Here's my go-to glossary of Teacher Conference Code Words and exactly what they mean.

Teacher Code Word #1: "Energetic"
Allow me to use it in a sentence (as Will's teacher did when I asked how things were going).

"Ohhhh, Will's my *energetic* little one in the mornings!"

Uh huh. I am not deceived. We all know this is doublespeak for "spastic," "bouncing off the walls," or maybe even, "Please, I beg of you, ask your doctor if Ritalin is right for you."

Teacher Code Word #2: "Demonstrates unwanted leadership skills"
This phrase was actually used *in real life* to describe my friend's daughter, and I've got to give the teacher props. This is the gentlest way

they've thought of yet to say, "This girl is bossy as hell, and she better simmer down before kids start raining wedgies upon her."

Teacher Code Word #3: "Exuberant" (or "Inquisitive")
Someone needs to level with you, so I guess it'll have to be Jackée.

Your kid is the one who will *not* put her hand down for two consecutive seconds, whose manic fervor to answer any and all questions is accompanied by intense straining and audible "Ooh ooh"s or "Me meee"s.

But before you start thinking that all this enthusiasm means you're the proud parent of a scholastic *wunderkind*, consider this: when the teacher finally calls on your kid, she's usually forgotten the question.

Teacher Code Word #4: "Social"
Your kid never stops talking. Ever. And he probably touches people a lot. Sometimes with boogers.

Teacher Code Word #5: "Disorganized"
I've learned the hard way that this is code for "blonde."

Your kid, like mine, lacks the wherewithal to turn in a signed permission slip or a check for the PTA pies or to bring home any one of her three lunch boxes. EVER. She leaves a trail of hat and mitten bread crumbs wherever she goes. She basically has no idea what is going on.

Teacher Code Word #6: "Does not apply himself" (or "Not living up to his full potential")
Sigh. This is the big one. This means your kid spaces out and thinks about Minecraft or Dippin' Dots or *anything but regrouping* and has downshifted into screensaver mode until recess when he can be free for ten whole minutes.

This is pretty much every kid.

Every so often, it is also procrastinating, mind-wandering, path-of-least-resistance *me*.

If I obsess over them too much, these conferences can send me into despair. I imagine every parent but me coming home with glowing reports like, "Wow, Mrs. Do-Right! I'm blown away at how your kid is applying himself like a boss!"

But I'm pretty sure nobody's hearing that. And if they *are* hearing that, that kid is probably raising his hand too much. And we've established that nobody likes that kid.

I know, I know, I know. We're not whipping out the flash cards enough or doing the bonus questions or going to Kumon or "Typing to Learn" or practicing viola twenty minutes a day.

There's no limit to all the things my kids could do if I only had it in me to run that show. All I know is that—*honestly and truly*—we are hitting it as hard as we can. And we're all *tired*.

As a mother, the reality is that I will never "live up to my full potential." No one ever does.

I may even "demonstrate unwanted leadership skills" from time to time.

I'll forever remain utterly "disorganized."

But at least no one would dare call me "energetic."

I will cling to that.

Purse: The Final Frontier
April 2012

"*Whew*! I can smell my purse!"

Those are words I actually said aloud. In a public place. In front of my child's teacher.

From the concerned looks I got, I might as well have shouted, "'Bout time to get rid of all these dead animal carcasses! They sho' nuf gettin' ripe!"

But knowing our way around the dark corners of a twenty-pound diaper bag like we do, we moms know that "Wooo! I can smell my purse" can mean any number of things. A mother's purse is a window into all she holds dear and needs close. Which, in this case, was a left-over chicken quesadilla.

I'd wisely saved it from lunch, wrapped all nice and tidy in greasy tin foil—all of it, except its Pepé Le Pew–like pungency.

On less stinky days, no one but me ever has to know what lies beneath—until I ended up at one of those buy-an-overpriced-monogrammed-utility-tote-or-we-won't-let-you-leave parties. (You know the kind.)

To break the ice (and the collective death grip on our wallets), the sales lady led us in a round of uncomfortable party games, including one that sent us digging through our pocketbooks to find stuff starting with certain letters.

Nice, normal things emerged from other people's bags.

"C" was for cell phone case in an adorable chevron pattern!

"P" was for pink nail polish in the perfect shade for summer toes!

But like a bad magician who misses the rabbit and pulls out a haddock, here's me . . . ta da . . . pulling out a week-old bottle of Happy Meal milk.

"M" for milk? Check.

Or better yet, how about "R" for rot? Or maybe "C" for chunks?

All this digging in bags and analyzing what's inside started to feel like taking a motherly inkblot test.

What does it say about me that I'd been carrying around a crappy box of cheapo crayons from that one time we ate at Chili's a year ago? Exhibited alongside a crumbly granola bar and a beat-up Fruit Roll-Up, I'd like to think it makes me a master of crisis management. (Although it probably has more to do with certain tendencies passed down by my ketchup packet–hoarding forebears.)

I also found some free-floating Tums and a half-eaten packet of Fun Dip, which demonstrate my healthy lifestyle.

There was also a bottle of hand sanitizer (for warding off evil spirits), a tin of Altoids (for post-quesadilla breath emergencies), and a month-old church bulletin (for making note of birthdays I'll feel guilty about never acknowledging).

On the bottom of my purse sat a sad pair of nineties-era sunglasses, scratched beyond repair and representative of how little I know of what's in style anymore. Bug eyes? *Risky Business*? Jackie O? No idea. I'll just squint.

Taken as a whole, my purse seems to say: I *try* to be prepared. I *try* to be thoughtful. I *try* to avoid illness and hunger and fashion victimhood.

I try.

But I also have dopey sunglasses, bad breath, and never enough snacks.

I fall short.

Surely I can't be alone in this. I must be just one mother out of millions like me, plodding along life's highway saddled with an oversized mom satchel full of linty lip balm, expired coupons, and maybe a touch of e-coli.

But let's look at the purse half-full, shall we?

No matter what the road brings, we never stop gunning for Mom of the Year. Every once in a while, we show up with curiously minty breath and well-fed children. And if we dig deep enough, we might even find enough loose change for a Coke.

Or better yet, on my very best day, a quesadilla.

As the World Turns
(and the Egg Timer Flies)
February 2010

I discovered I wasn't the person I thought I was the moment I launched an egg timer into the living room wall.

It was one of those motherly moments of blind fury—a moment in which there were no words left in the English language to talk sense into my unreasonable male child.

So I did it. I launched the nearest throwable thing across the room at full force. My throwing arm's not much, but still, the timer was reduced to plastic rubble. (I blame China.)

After I swept the collection of plastic parts into the trash, I tried to turn it into a punch line.

"Better the egg timer than Will," I fake laughed. But I don't need to tell you—it's a scene I wasn't proud of.

Because until I saw that ridiculous egg timer hurtle at Mach 10 from my clinched fist, I honestly never thought I had it in me. I guess no parent ever does.

———————

Before I had kids, I could have sworn I was a happy, calm, well-adjusted human being. Day in and day out, I could somehow cope with five-alarm work stress and infuriating coworkers without hurling the first insult or paperweight.

Looking back now, I might have suffered from just a touch of Mary Poppins Syndrome. I seemed to think I was "practically perfect in every way."

Then God gave me my firstborn son.

Bull-headed, armed with an argument for *everything*, Will was born with the codes for pushing all my buttons.

But in all my daily struggles to be "good," motherhood has managed to shine a light on the true content of my character—some of it fine and loving, some of it harsh, shrill, and just plain ugly. It's given me a far clearer (albeit less flattering) picture of who I really am deep down inside. And let's just say, it's not always my best side.

But if I'm ever going to start weeding out the nasty bits, knowing that junk's in there must be at least a *quarter* of the battle, right?

Still, all this screaming into pillows and throwing stuff—it gets loud and exhausting and *old*. At its core, it's just not good government policy, so Will's kindergarten teacher gave me another strategy to try. (Oh, I have a new one every week.)

There's a name for it and a book about it, but it boils down to swift justice—just nipping stuff in the bud and not *talking* the kid to death. Thus, the child has been in an almost constant state of "time out" lately. This approach has been met with much arm-flapping, shrieking, and victimized sobbing. ("But I didn't do anything wronnnng!")

This is what causes housewives to drink before noon. And throw things.

My favorite of these whimsical scenes was the day Will was dragged into time-out kicking, screaming, and stupidly calling me "stupid."

"I didn't mean to say you were stupid!" he backpeddled wildly. "I just meant to say you were *ignorant*!"

Now you know I had to write that one down. Not only is that hilarious, but, *oh man*, it's the God's honest truth.

Sure, I've got enough book learning to spell *antidisestablishmentarianism* (just don't ask me what it *is*), but nothing in this world lets you know you are miles out of your depth like trying to raise another human being into civilized adulthood.

In fact, if parenting has taught me anything, it's how little I know—and how far I have to go.

So thanks for the daily life lesson, kid, which goes something like this: "Ugh, I screwed up. I really need to work on that. Ugh, I screwed up. I need to work on that some more. Ugh, I screwed up. Where are more books that I won't read about this topic?" You get the idea.

Now, sweet child, since we've established that we're both still works in progress, will you please, in the name of all things holy and pure, stop giving me all this lip and go to bed?

If you won't do it for me, please, *I beg of you.*

Do it for the egg timer.

My Resolutions for a "Good Enough" Year

January 2008

I usually make a resolution not to make resolutions (since those set up a nice little tradition of failure I'd rather just avoid).

But this year, I was thinking if I made my resolutions bite-sized enough—rather than the usual sweeping pronouncements about being a better wife, mother, and citizen of the world—maybe I could experience the joy of actually checking some off.

I give you, then, this mother's official New Year's resolutions (not necessarily in order of importance).

1. *I will try not to groan so much.* At the littlest things my kids do, I find myself sighing with the dramatic flourish of a silent-screen star. I groan, slump, and roll my eyes heavenwards a million times a day, usually over dumb stuff like the sound of Honeycombs crunching into the carpet or Will taking off all his clothes to use the toilet. Not only are these things not a big deal, but they're sometimes kind of funny. I should just laugh at the joke now and then.

2. *I will try to look* at *my children, not* through *them.* When they're talking, playing, living, I want to be more in the moment—instead of constantly rearranging my mental checklist.

3. *I will try to look* at *my husband, not* through *him.* (See #2.) And when he looks back at me, I'd like to occasionally be wearing makeup and a clean shirt.

4. *I will try to stop worrying about having all these deeply enriching parent-child experiences using Popsicle sticks or egg cartons.* When caught up in the pressure to craft, I'll spend all morning orchestrating a project with much hovering and carping over what *not* to do with the Magic Markers. Five minutes later, Will inevitably wanders off bored and henpecked, leaving me fuming in a tiny chair. Fast-forward to me stomping over to the TV to turn on whatever PBS is showing, even if it means Barney. We'd all be far less damaged if I'd just sit and watch him play with his trains and fake like I'm interested.

5. *I will try not to bow and scrape to my kids' demands.* They've both got two healthy (albeit short) legs, and it's my job to start teaching them to fetch their own stuff and pick up their own messes.

6. *I will try to get a babysitter more often than each Olympiad.*

7. *I will try to clean the bathroom before there are visible signs of fungal growth.*

8. *I will try to get to the dentist.* I haven't had a cleaning since the B.C. (before-children) years. My yellowing incisors have been fondly dubbed "the corn niblets." Time to shine.

9. *I will try to put a few pictures from Lucy's young life in an album.* I will not use craft scissors or hole punches or join a scrapbooking cult. But I will try to document that she actually exists in an album—instead of in that leaning tower of photo sleeves on our hall shelf.

10. *I will try to remember the quote on my fridge that says, "There is no way to be a perfect mother, but a million ways to be a good one."*

This year, above all, I'll try to be a good mom—and a basically contented one. Even if I'm up to my yellowing eyeteeth in imperfections.

Birthday Cake
with a Side of Crow
February 2009

I love the taste of crow in the morning. It goes great with birthday cake.

Let's just say my disdain for overblown kiddie birthday parties has been shouted from the hilltops more than a few times. I've called jumpy-castle-sized affairs a big fat waste of money, a feeble attempt to keep up with the Joneses, and a heaping helping of unhealthy adulation on kids who won't remember any of it. I pretty much still feel that way.

But did those feelings stop me from marching down to the local indoor playground, tossing them my wallet, and begging them to be my surrogate party planner?

Nope, they did not.

Because Will is turning five this month, and the child is obsessed with having the perfect non-family/all-the-school-friends party. He has literally spent the last eleven months going over the invitation list. He's worked up party themes well into puberty (though something tells me he'll ditch the construction site cake scheduled for birthday fourteen).

The kid is fighting for his right to party.

Meanwhile, I've spent the past year toying with all kinds of sleight-of-hand tricks—birthday trips as a family to big-city museums, kid-friendly eateries, outer space—anything entertaining that doesn't require an *actual* party with live children in our postage stamp–sized house.

(I should note that, in our case, size *does* matter. Our house has roughly the same dimensions as a Hobbit's hovel under a tree stump.

We *can* stand upright in here, but there's zero flapping room for the Funky Chicken.)

But there's a bigger fear afoot.

I read *Lord of the Flies* in high school. I know that when seemingly cherubic youngsters get together, mass hysteria spreads, turning them into something akin to Walmart crazies at the dawning of Black Friday.

I can just picture them all pouring into my house, tying me up with party streamers, and surrounding me with demands of fun, sugar, and something to bounce upon. My only defense will be some boring homemade games involving fishing poles with dangling paper clips.

As if in a nightmare, I can hear myself trying to announce (with the sweetness of a June Cleaver and the unquestioned authority of a General Patton): "Everyone gather 'round so we can all make a fun dinosaur hat!"

But just like in my nightmares, when I try to scream, no sound comes out. There I stand, mute and impotent, with rabid preschoolers spinning around my legs, pursuing each other with hot vengeance and clunking each other with my own handcrafted fishing poles. Next thing you know, my head's being mounted on the neighbor's lamppost.

I know when I'm in over my head (while it's still attached).

So this year, since Will's only five and I'm already too old, I am publicly crying uncle. For once, I'm recognizing my limits, and I'm phoning it in.

I'll do my motherly duty and show up with dinosaur cupcakes and goodie bags filled with (spoiler alert) tiny capsules that balloon into T-Rexes when you add water. But then I'll just set that marauding band of boys loose and watch the ensuing mayhem through the camcorder lens from a comfortable chair—one that's nowhere near my living room.

Every other day of the year, Will gets to hear me hollering "Hurry up!" or "Stop climbing on the furniture!" or "Eat that blasted chicken nugget before Jesus comes back!" But just this once, I'm going to try putting down the mom megaphone in favor of sitting back and enjoying the party.

Some days, the saner, sweeter thing for everybody is to stop trying to make magic happen. Some days, it's just showing up—and really being there.

Uncle. And hallelujah.

Welcome to the Breakfast Club
August 2014

This past spring, I drove eight hundred miles back home to North Carolina to sit by my mother's bedside during her last days.

There was nothing much to do but sit with my siblings and my dad and watch it happen, nibble on cheese and crackers, make awkward chit-chat with visitors, and sometimes try to tell her things I thought she should know. It was grueling. But when we stepped outside those nursing home doors, nobody knew our mother was dying. Especially not that girl at the Popeye's drive-thru.

One of those grim mornings, my sister and I had the bright idea to pick up some chicken biscuits—you know, to help gird our loins. We were pretty sure this would be Mom's last day. We'd need protein and something deep-fried to get through it.

But I promise you have never sat in a drive-thru line so excruciatingly long in all your livelong days. And you have never met a slower, more spaced-out drive-thru worker in the history of drive-thru workers (and that's saying something). I'm talking *glacial*. While we waited for her to pluck the chicken bald, the most awful gallows humor kicked in. We started thinking up the cheeriest, most horrifying things we wanted to say to this poor woman—all in our sweetest, most singsong Southern way, of course.

Things like, "No, really . . . it's *okay*! We've got *nothing* better to do. Our mother is only on her *deathbed*. In fact, she could very well be knocking on the pearly gates right this very minute. But we'd rather miss our mother's passing any day of the week than miss those biscuits! So really and truly, you just take your sweet time, dear! We'll *wait*!"

We went on and on like that until the tears were streaming and our fists were hammering the dashboard. It's safe to say we were a little unhinged.

That drive-thru girl had no idea who she was dealing with that day—or what we were dealing with. *You just never know.*

And I think nowadays it's harder to know.

We only know what we see from photos online—usually filtered, scenic, and all smiles. Most of us tend to put the good stuff out there and hold the bad stuff close to the chest. I don't have a problem with that, exactly. I mean, I love the good stuff—like cute pictures of your kids (and I hope you can tolerate mine).

But since we're all putting our prettiest selves out there for public consumption—and since little nibbles of electronic conversation often count as "connection"—we don't always know what's behind the curtain of each beautiful life. And there's a lot.

If I hadn't actually talked about this stuff in real life with these people, I would have never known the smiling young couple traipsing across Europe had just lost their first baby. I wouldn't have known the lovely college girl with the impeccable wardrobe was battling a painful mystery illness, or the happy family at the beach had just clawed their way back from adultery.

Way down in the depths that Instagram can't see, you just never know what's *really* going on with people. Down there, everyone is a mess. *Everyone.* And the parts that aren't a mess are only display-worthy because of the handiwork of God's merciful mending kit.

We are the Breakfast Club—each of us a brain, an athlete (maybe not so much), a basket case, a princess, and a criminal. No matter what we look like to the world outside, we are all a confounding mess. Every last one of us. And we all need grace—and each other.

So that woman you see doubled over laughing at the drive-thru? She could be on her way to a loved one's deathbed. (If she is, that would be really weird. But believe me, it could happen.)

What she'd want more than anything is for you to give her a big smile and a bag full of biscuits.

Just make it snappy.

PART II

CRISES DU JOUR

Menus from roadside diners are, to me, the highest form of origami (if there was actually such a thing as laminated origami featuring photos of lamb gyros).

There's just *so much folding* involved. Diner choices are so plentiful, it takes half an hour just to unfold and unflap this abundant accordion—only to discover in amazement there's *even more on the back*.

I always marvel how one kitchen could hold enough ingredients and know-how to pull this off. I mean, those guys in the kitchen have to be "game on" every single day; they never know what's coming.

I could order the borscht or the chocolate chip pancakes. This day could go any which way.

Parenting is kind of like that.

One day could end in a bike wipe-out with a side of scabs.

Another day could bring a steaming pile of homework tears, friend drama, and grass stains followed by a palate cleanser of adorable homemade daisy chains.

Another day might serve up a buffet of boneless temper tantrums, last-minute science projects, missed naps, and blanket forts topped off with an impromptu afternoon of couch snuggles.

Who knows? Today might be the day for the dreaded principal call or the midnight puke-fest or maybe even the winning goal you never thought you'd live to see.

As parents, we never know what each day will bring—what joys or sorrows or papier-mâché volcanoes might explode upon our lives. (I've written about a lot of those moments in this section.)

But somehow we parents have to be ready (or *get* ready fast) for all of it—with a bucket or a Band-Aid or a bear hug or a nice long teary bedtime prayer.

The world could serve up anything today, moms and dads of the world—some of it delicious, some of it heartburn-inducing, sometimes both at once.

As for me and my house, we will order the chocolate chip pancakes. Preferably with a side of thick-cut bacon.

The day could go either way. I feel it's important to be prepared.

Lost: One Stuffed Dog
and All My Marbles

Author's note: This sweet little crisis is where it all began. This is the second-ever Tales from the Crib *column, published October 2, 2007. (The first-ever was like most first-evers . . . a little shaky and wobbly.) Since then, at least a jillion more words have spilled onto paper about my poor, beloved, defenseless children. Will and Lucy, I'm sorry. I love you to pieces, but you just give me so. Much. Fodder.*

It was bound to happen, and today was the day. My three-year-old, Will, lost his favorite stuffed puppy, Casey, at the mall.

But let me state up front before you get too mournful (because you *know* what a Code Red situation this is): *We have found the dog.*

I'm rejoicing to have learned that Will's BFF is squatting at babyGap until we can get back to claim him. But let me tell you, it was one heck of a sickening feeling to realize we'd returned home today *sans chien.* Thankfully, one frantic phone call gave me the happy news that Casey is in the Gap's custody, safe and sound and still sheathed in the diaper Will wrapped around him this morning.

This news was small comfort to a small boy whose ever-present sidekick was nowhere near his side. The tears were overflowing, the wailing was deafening, and if he could've reached the pedals, I believe he would have commandeered the Volvo for an emergency rescue mission himself.

Named for a neighborhood dog that Will adored, Casey was intended to be "Will's gift" to his newborn baby sister. But as soon as I bought it, I knew my cutesy idea was naive. Will immediately began transferring his affections (as Jane Austen would put it) from the bear/blanket hybrid he'd dragged around for his first two years of life to this new, fluffier friend. He basically stole the dog from his unsuspecting lump of a sister.

Now Casey is Will's softest, plushest appendage. When something funny makes us all laugh, Will runs to find Casey so he/she (the pronoun is ever-changing) won't miss it. When Will's excited to greet someone, he tosses Casey with glee in the unsuspecting friend's direction. When Will is in a fit of oral fixation, he chews furiously on Casey's ever-flattening nose.

He's abused this poor animal with such rough affection that I have to keep re-stitching Casey's floppy neck to keep its head from completely falling off.

Needless to say, Casey is on the must-have list for every outing, nap, and waking moment. And of course, Casey has been dropped somewhere along the way on just about every one of those outings—thankfully remembered (by me) and retrieved (by me) before all was lost.

So now the debate begins. Should we seek a Casey *doppelgänger*? Or would a stand-in be viewed with only suspicion, and ultimately, rejection? Does Gund even *make* this thing anymore? These are critical issues to discuss around the family dinner table tonight.

All I know is I don't want to be there when Casey goes missing for real. We might just become the first family desperate enough to post a stuffed animal's furry face on the side of a milk carton.

The Tale of the Prodigal Tooth Fairy

November 2011

Candidates vying for Mother of the Year do not wake up to the words *Mommy, the Tooth Fairy didn't come.*

Nothing kicks a fuzzy morning brain into guilty high gear like four sad, gigantic eyes staring at you from your bedside, wondering why everything wondrous they believed to be true is a lie.

That'll wake you up. And break your heart.

I sat up bolt-straight at those words, staring at my children with the darting eyes of the hunted (and the half asleep), my mouth hanging open dumbly.

As they filled me in on all the injurious details, it came flooding back—the "oh yeah" of remembering last night's lost tooth and the "aw nuts" of remembering how completely I'd forgotten it.

"It almost makes me think," Will said pointedly, "that somebody comes and takes my tooth, puts a dollar under my pillow, and just throws my tooth in the garbage."

(Yeah, well, that pretty much covers it.)

As he floated that trial balloon with quiet brokenness, he might as well have been Dennis Franz slamming me against the precinct wall. I nearly spilled my guts right then and there.

Oh, he had me.

But then, as if guided by the magical powers of the fairy realms, I hatched a plan. (Some might call it another lie; I call it a *plan*.)

I sent Will and Lucy off to tell Daddy their tale of woe while I returned to the scene of the crime. As soon as those little backs were turned (try imagining this in cinematic slow motion), I grabbed a crumpled dollar from last night's jeans pocket and flung it onto the floor near their bunk bed.

My new lie (I mean, *plan*) was proclaimed: "Behold! The Tooth Fairy has come indeed! Her gift merely *fell* from your pillow in the night!"

As I internally congratulated my quick thinking, the boy genius pointed out a small hole in my story.

The tooth was still under his pillow.

Good point. Time for lie number two. (Or was it lie number three? I've lost count).

Seeing Will's favorite stuffed dog perched next to the bunk ladder, I grasped like a mad man at straws and new lies—proposing that maybe, just maybe, his completely unmenacing, unmoving, cuddly-wuddly stuffed dog had scared off the Tooth Fairy before she could grab the goods.

I know. It was a total load of hooey.

I can't believe it actually worked.

Next thing I know, we were back to happily discussing how the Tooth Fairy must use pixie dust to shrink dollar bills for ease of transport and other fairy logistics.

Crisis averted . . . for now.

———————

Some say it's wrong to fill children's heads with falsehoods and fantasies. My response to that philosophy is one of great depth and thoughtfulness.

Ba-lo-ney.

Nobody ends up popping Prozac because Daddy lied about reindeer on the roof.

Filling a home with intangibles like imagination and playfulness (sometimes fueled by a healthy dose of tall tales) is, to me, an act of love.

Children's brains are wonderfully wired this way, and I intend to keep up the charade as long as they'll let me.

Or until they read this.

Or until yours do and tell mine about it.

Oh brother, maybe you should just tear out these pages and swallow/burn/let the bird poop on them.

We're all in this great big happy conspiracy together. I won't crack if you won't.

Answering the Big Questions of Life, Death, and Where Babies Come From (or Not . . .)

January 2010

"Mom, what was it like . . ."

My ears perked up like a couple of those satellite dishes searching for signs of extraterrestrial life. (It isn't often my kindergartener thinks outside of his Will-sized box, so when he does, I'm all big ears and eye contact.)

". . . to have a baby come out of you?"

Oh, sweet Jesus. I did *not* see that one coming.

Between all the frenzied heart palpitations and my need to buy time, I slowly pulled up a chair and started searching for my most evasive vocabulary words. Not sure what he was driving at, I decided to go for something akin to honesty.

"Well, it hurts," I said. "But the doctors help you. And our bodies are designed so it all works just like it's supposed to."

That last statement was issued with such happy finality, I thought surely he'd accept these vagaries as gospel and move on. He did not.

"But how does it come out?" he insisted. "How do you get it *out*?"

Now, let me explain a bit about myself that you would probably figure out after five minutes in my presence: I'm a total prude. I'm squeamish about all things fleshly. There's a very real possibility I was born in a turtleneck.

As such, I've never felt led to instruct my young children on the anatomically correct names for every darn nook and cranny of the human body. It may sound backward to you, but I'm seriously skeeved by toddlers these days who go around talking about everybody's naughty bits like the girls of *Sex and the City*.

So when pressed on the mechanics of childbirth, I girded my puritanical loins, then cringed and staggered into uncharted territory.

"Well, it's not like pooping exactly," I said. (I *know*. It's so horrifying, I'm embarrassed to write it.) "But the baby comes out *down there*."

I stared expectantly at him with this weird Cheshire Cat grin on my face—one meant to implore, "Okay, does that do it? Can we be done talking about this now?"

He looked up into my sweaty face with relief.

"Oh, that's good," he said. Then he hoisted some sort of imaginary weapon over his head. "They could have killed me if they'd used an axe."

I laughed so hard I nearly split the seams of my granny panties.

————————

Feeling my way through these out-of-the-blue, heart-to-heart inquisitions feels a bit like being a contestant on *$25,000 Pyramid*.

Without warning, my kids will hand me a card with some lofty concept on it (Reproduction! The Afterlife! Why Darth Vader Chose Evil!), and suddenly it's my job to pepper them with clues to the meaning of life without using any of the big words.

It's one of the parenting challenges I secretly love.

And it's a good thing, because four-year-old Lucy just roped me into a doozy.

It seems that, without my even realizing it, she'd soaked up a lot of words around here lately about my ailing mother and nursing homes and friends dying young.

So one night, warm from the tub and wrapped in a towel in my arms, she whimpered, "I don't want to die."

Oh, she'd heard too much.

For the next half hour, as I tucked her into her flannel sheets with the dancing fairies on them, I tried everything.

I offered well-worn platitudes. "Sweetie, you've got *years* of life ahead of you!"

I tried happy endings. Me: "We have a better place to look forward to!" Lucy: "Maybe, but they won't have my bed there!"

Nothing worked. All I did was tangle myself into big fat knots trying to explain how her stuffed giraffe can't die since, well, it's not *technically* alive (a filthy lie, she protested) or how when someone dies, they can't be with us anymore. ("But I'll miss you!" she wailed.) The whole conversation was almost too much for us both to bear.

There's just no way—then or ever—that I'll get all her questions of life and death answered, all neat and tidy.

But I did all I knew to do for one night. I held her tight. I sang her a lullaby or three. And I told her about heaven.

For good measure, so did her brother, who chimed in from the top bunk in all his hard-earned wisdom: "But Lucy, heaven's a beautiful place. And they'll have Legos!"

I'm sure glad one of us seems to have all the answers.

Pilgrims, Indians, and the Pickiest Child in the New World

November 2007

This Thanksgiving, our family did what normal American families do. We ate ourselves into a whole new weight category.

At least, three of the four of us did. Our three-year-old ate yogurt.

No Stove Top. No pumpkin pie. Just *yogurt*.

Now before you get all judgy, please note that there was some wheat germ swirled in to make me think it was extra nutritious (and sprinkles on top to make Will think it wasn't).

I'd dotted his plate with the obligatory shreds of turkey and company, but I wasn't fooling anybody. I knew it was little more than a future offering to the garbage can gods.

I am the proud parent of the pickiest child alive.

I already know your next question. No, he won't eat peanut butter, hot dogs, or mac and cheese. His is a repertoire countable on two hands—dominated by processed chicken nuggets that bear no resemblance to actual poultry.

Will has always tormented his father and me at dinner hour. Not only would he not want the food we'd place on his high-chair tray, but he'd hand it right back. He didn't even want it entering his airspace.

More recently, we had a showdown I now lovingly refer to as "the string cheese incident."

It started with his simple but surprising request for a cheese stick. Even though I'd tried to foist cheese sticks on him countless times before, I, like other mothers, cling to hope and the annoying mantra that kids may have to be presented with a new food ten times before they'll try it. (I highly doubt parents in Ethiopia need these strategies, but that's another topic for another day.).

I knew in my motherly heart of hearts that he'd never eat it, but I made him swear on his favorite stuffed animal's life that he would. He crossed his heart, then promptly tore off a shred of cheese . . . not to *eat* it, mind you. Don't be ridiculous.

No, his plan was to hollow out his cheese stick into a boat perfect for toting his other uneaten foodstuffs.

Impotent rage swelled within. I asked myself, "What would Dr. Phil do?" Then I locked myself into a deal with the Devil. My child would *not* leave that table until he ate at least one teeny-tiny string from that blankety-blank stick of cheese.

This was a deal I'd live to regret (which is how most alliances with Satan tend to go).

An hour later, picture me, neck muscles bulging, screeching from across the kitchen, "Oh. My. Lord. It's a piece of cheese, not a shrink-wrapped *turd*!"

Pearls of wisdom indeed.

He finally choked down the cheese, probably because he'd finally had enough of being on the receiving end of my crazy eyes.

(Meanwhile, picture two-year-old Lucy popping pearl onions in her mouth as her parents swoon with love.)

Except for overly energetic approaches like sneaking broccoli purées into his barbeque sauce or fashioning his food into smiley faces, I swear we've tried it all.

We've tried stern. "No getting down until you've eaten these micro-scopic bites of pork chop." Parental seething ensues.

We've tried breezy. "If you don't want to eat, fine. But the kitchen's closed." Worrying about iron deficiencies ensues.

We've tried "no-thank-you bites" where he must at least *try* every-thing on his plate. Gagging ensues.

We've bribed. We've been short-order cooks. Now we're back to being stern with a twist of bitter.

People insist that one day he'll eat us out of house and home. Maybe.

Or maybe he'll just be the annoying guest at your dinner party one day who says, "Oh, sorry. I don't like nuts . . . Velveeta . . . iceberg lettuce." (Swap those out with any normal food of your choice).

We're certainly hoping for better, but we've been burned before.

So if Will does show up at your house scrounging for food, just point him to the nearest Burger King.

I hear special orders don't upset them.

The Chronicles of Nausea
January 2008

It's a classic tale, but a tragic one.

Girl meets microbe. Girl licks microbe. Microbe tap dances up and down girl's intestinal tract.

Girl pukes. Girl pukes on many things she shouldn't. Girl pukes some more.

Mom lathers, scrubs, launders, detoxifies, rinses, and repeats.

Brother meets microbe. Mom and Dad meet microbe. Gruesome cycle is continued until marauding microbe runs out of victims.

Heaven help us. Our family is just emerging from the nuclear winter of the stomach flu.

Everyone I've talked to this holiday season has a jolly tale of a yuletide laid waste by nausea, and we were no exception. The difference is that we drove two days and nearly a thousand miles to take our turn.

The entire week after Christmas while visiting family down South, we fell like dominos in front of my mother-in-law's toilet, one by one by one by one. It wasn't pretty. I personally wanted to die for a few bleak hours—time that, by rights, should have been spent catching up on all the deep-fried Southern delicacies I'd been hankering for all year long.

But with our stomachs in sudden revolt against all foods but saltines, Maurice's Piggie Park was out of the question. (Unless you've experienced a Little Joe basket with hushpuppies, you can't know what a cruel disappointment that is.)

And I'll just be real honest. When it comes to all that scares me most in life, the stomach bug is right up there with *Children of the Corn* and two-piece swimsuits.

From that first awful moment when Lucy woke up sick, I was scared I'd get it (I did); scared Will would get it (*he* did—at the Sheraton on our trip back for bonus fun); scared of where or on whom they'd get sick (the backseat of the car was my personal favorite); scared to let the sickly ones drink anything; scared of them ending up in the ER because I'd been too scared to let them drink anything. I was haunted by a vile population of microscopic menaces. I couldn't see them, but I knew they were there. Hiding. Multiplying. Plotting their attack.

Funny how it's the things we *can't* see that scare us most—monsters under the bed, murderers behind the bushes, kidney stones, and that paramecium death squad I imagined lurking on every doorknob, light switch, and square inch of the bathroom linoleum.

In my mind, they'd become those black demonic shadows in *Ghost*, galloping around the rim of the toilet bowl, festering in the Lego box, teeming in the carpet fibers. If I could've borrowed a black light from *Dateline*, I was convinced their evil presence would have lit up the room like a Lite-Brite (with *You're next* spelled out in a sinister glow).

For all I know, those foul beasts are doing the can-can right here on my seat cushion.

At some point, you just have to let it go. You eventually have to lay down your arms and your Lysol and just be grateful you made it through alive; be grateful that this illness was just a rocky patch, not our daily cross to bear; be grateful that what had seemed like endless misery is already a distant memory.

Or at least it will be—once I burn every last one of Lucy's germ-infested stuffed animals.

It's for the best, don't you think?

I'm sure she'll thank me for it later.

A Tale of Two Potties
July 2008

Warning: The following includes references to poop and other gross stuff. Watch your step.

———————

It all started with Lucy backing up to the bushes in our yard, hiking up her shirt (with her diaper still on), and informing us she was "going potty." It must've seemed the thing to do after watching her brother fire away at whatever rock, shrub, or body of water he deemed worthy.

Now Lucy, at two and a half, is regularly insisting she needs to go. And get this . . . she actually *goes*. In the potty. After which, we squeal and dance around the output like it's a gift from the gods.

Sorry, but I'm just a wee bit ecstatic. I never believed it could be so easy—not after all our boy child put us through.

———————

Exactly one year ago, when Will was three and a half (and about to outgrow the biggest Pampers they make), I decided it was time. (Way past time, actually.) After a million false starts, we just had to quit fiddle-farting around and make this potty-training thing stick.

No waffling. No caving. No going back.

Predictably, Will did not agree.

In the process, he nearly drove his dear mother to early morning drinking and a frontal lobotomy. (I could actually *feel* my personalities splitting some days.)

One moment, I'd be springing with glee into the ceiling fan blades at the sight of a turd in a bowl. The next moment, I'd be hissing, "Are you doing this to torture me?" as I removed the afternoon's fifth pair of saturated Thomas the Tank Engine skivvies.

The only thing getting flushed around here was my self-esteem.

I'll admit right up front: if you're reading this and you breathe in and out, you would have to be a better potty trainer than me.

Even if you've never had a toddler, a guinea pig, or so much as a sea monkey, it doesn't matter. You'd be better than me. Trust me on this. I flunked out of every potty-training school of thought one by one.

I tried it Supernanny-style, complete with chart and stickers.

I offered incentive packages—everything from Popsicles to ponies.

I heaped praise.

I read books.

I tried not to throw things.

Then the day came when the final straw snapped (helped along by a rushing torrent of pee). Will had insisted he didn't need to go when we got off that highway exit in search of fast food. Though he claimed to be in perfect control of that wee bladder, he still managed *somehow* to gully wash the entire restaurant booth *and* my husband's shorts that fine day.

That's the moment it all hit the fan. But from then on, "it" didn't hit anywhere else (if you catch my not-so-subtle drift).

The kid finally got it. He got it the hard way, but he got it.

———————

Now enter Lucy a year later in angel wings, training herself all on her own initiative. I've had absolutely nothing to do with it.

So here's what I'm thinking: if I only play a small part in Lucy's success story, then maybe I can let myself off the hook a little for Will's epic struggle.

It's obvious I had no idea what I was doing with Will, and I still don't with Lucy. But she's just showing me yet again how wildly different two children can be and how sometimes what they choose to do (or refuse to do) isn't *entirely* a reflection on my parenting.

When I start believing it's all me, I give myself way too much credit—and sometimes too much blame. Because no matter how many Dum Dums I dangled, Will never budged without a fight. Yet, here's Lucy, ready for the big-girl pants without the first mention of a reward.

So I've stumbled onto something obvious to everyone but me—that my children aren't pint-sized robots to be programmed. They're two very different people, responding to challenges in very different ways.

Not exactly a news flash, but still somehow liberating.

So I suppose whether they buck and kick or go willingly, my charge is to lead these little horses to water the best I can and just pray they'll drink.

Or in Lucy's case, pee. And preferably not on my husband.

Fall is Another Word
for Face-Plant
September 2010

I'm not sure who that stupid jerk Murphy is, but his law was bound to kick in sooner or later. Back-to-school was going a little *too* smoothly.

Launching into our first week of school, I put on the bus two of the most cheerful little kids ever bound for elementary school.

The night before her first day of kindergarten, Lucy had peeked out from the covers and whispered she was scared, that she wished she could be in her big brother's first-grade class instead. But once Day One dawned, she showed the world nothing but miles of teeth gleaming through the smudgy bus window.

(Her mother, on the other hand, showed the world a blubbering mess. Nothing a morning of mimosas with my kindergarten mom friends couldn't fix.)

The kids came home happy. They went back the next day happy. They had no happy-killing homework. Better yet, I had three straight happy hours all to myself.

Happy, happy, happy.

I should have seen it coming.

Had I learned nothing from my years of *Guiding Light* training? I should have known by now that giddy happiness is the ultimate foreshadower. Whenever a favorite once-dead character is resurrected from a fiery car crash to rekindle lost love, you better brace yourself for the evil twin. The happy just can't last.

So I should've heard the time bomb ticking when Will stepped off the bus after Day Four with both shoes—as usual—*untied.*

I'm so used to this being his shoes' permanent condition ("Once tied, always tied" is his philosophy) that I didn't even bother pestering him. I figured he'd mastered the fine art of navigating those dangling laces, forgetting that the kid is Dick Van Dyke incarnate, tripping over every ottoman in his path.

Sure enough, no sooner had he crossed the threshold than his laces got wedged under the shutting door, and the kid went down. Hard. Face-first into an end table.

There was blood and sobbing and breathless calls to the pediatrician—three things in life I can seriously do without.

Fast-forward to my little boy, flat on his back at the doctor's office, wailing and curling his toes as six stitches knit his soft, sweet, baby-face back together again. It wasn't pretty, and the kindest nurse ever told me not to look. But I couldn't help it. I peeked.

While I death-gripped his little hands, while he tried to be brave but begged for it to stop, this is where I started to check out. Will was the one being poked with needles, yet I was the pathetic one sweating and teetering and hearing a freight train in my ears, who had to sit down while the nurse yelled at me to put my head between my knees.

It was one of those primal motherly experiences, something on paper that shouldn't be that awful, but it was.

My child was in pain, I couldn't make it stop, and my world (and the room) started spinning. It was as basic as that.

He's fixed up beautifully now, self-conscious about his temporary Frankenstein look but no worse for the wear. Still, as my wise friend with a grown-up son reminded me, "Little kids, little problems. Big kids, big problems."

So we got off to a great start, we hit a snag, and we stitched him back up again.

Good as new.

I can only pray that all life's bumps can be so neatly patched together again. But something tells me I better get out my smelling salts—just in case.

One Heck of a
Hare-Brained Scheme

December 2011

I can pinpoint the exact moment I realized we weren't ready to be dog people.

It happened when the pound puppy I'd gone to meet introduced herself by piddling on the floor and then lapping it up like it was Mountain Dew.

The animal control lady was standing right there sizing up my dog owner potential, so I mustered my best game face as though—tra la la!—this kind of stuff happens all the time at our house.

(A lot of weird stuff does go on there, but Lord have mercy, not that.)

I'd gone to the shelter thinking we were all-in for a dog, but that pee-drinking business scared me straight. I left there all-in for a cat.

But of course, there's the small problem of my cat-adverse husband. Nothing can convince him to share his airspace with a feline.

Yet we've got two animal-loving kids in our house who've been foaming at the mouth for a pet *since birth*. In fact, our nearly-six-year-old, Lucy, had informed me that all she wanted for her birthday this year was "something live."

We first tried to pacify this animal lust with a betta fish. Swimming under a layer of dusty sludge, Shiny now warrants little more than a passing glance and the occasional wish that he'd sprout legs and a personality.

Fish—check. Cat—nope. Dog—maybe later. Seems we were running out of "live" options.

Snakes and lizards were non-starters . . . for obvious reasons.

I'd done my time with gerbils. Not only are they boring, but I can't purge that cedar shaving smell from my childhood memories.

Someone even suggested a ferret. But to me, ferrets are the dirty old men of the animal kingdom; they strike me as the greasiest and most unsavory of characters.

Then one fateful day, some friends told us about a lop-eared bunny they'd had—not in a hutch, but actually *in their house*. He'd had a little cage, but he mostly chillaxed on the rug while they watched TV.

This was a revelation—people did this?

The closest I'd seen was a girl who walked her rabbit on a leash. Wacky as that was, this was something even more radical. A rabbit hanging around the house—sort of like a dog that never barks and never drinks its own pee? It might be just weird enough to work.

I started googling the heck out of our little cotton-tailed friends ... and Shazam! We now have Edna.

Edna was the name she was given at the rabbit rescue (again, who knew there was such a thing?) since apparently she's no spring chick. But the name made us laugh, and so does the fact that we now have a white bunny with gray spots. In our house.

Will repeats daily, "It's like a dream, Mom. We have a bunny!"

That it is. Man, oh man, the things we do for our kids. So now when Lucy gets home from school, she darts right past me, squealing "Edna!" (at a volume I'm sure rabbits love). Then she grabs a stack of books to "read" to the bunny while rubbing roughly at the poor creature's ears.

You can't help but picture Bugs Bunny in the vice grip of the big red monster, getting the daylights squeezed out of him with pure love.

I hope Edna enjoys the works of Seuss and having lettuce shoved in her face.

Because that's love, Lucy-style.

And apart from bunny suicide by gnawed power cords, that love is here to stay. In our house.

I guess this is what happens when you love the daylights out of someone.

Author's Note: *We are now also dog people. Oh, and there's a second fish. And if you can believe it, a cat. The menagerie grows ...*

The Lesson of the Lazarus Fish
January 2012

It's a Christmas miracle.

Against all odds, we made it through the holidays with both kids a) still believing in Santa even after dear ol' dad let it slip that he'd ordered those Nerf guns from Amazon, and b) still believing that the fish in the bowl is their pet, Shiny. (Which he is not. He is a blatant fraud.)

Let me back up. There's clearly more to this story.

As we prepared for our Christmas travels, I'd recruited a neighbor girl to watch our new bunny, Edna. I'd left her copious notes. There'd even been a training session. And then I remembered—duh, we also have a fish.

Thankfully, Shiny's daily regimen boiled down to one word: pellet. That critter was indestructible. Or so I thought.

Eight days in, I got a call from the girl's mom, invoking the tone of a school nurse with bad news.

"Everything's *fine* with Edna!" she exclaimed. "She's doing *just great*!" (More details followed of just how perfectly fantabulous the rabbit was.)

Then came the subject she clearly dreaded. Shiny, it seemed, had begun the tell-tale side-flop of a fish circling life's drain. They would be happy to pick up a spare, she insisted, *if* we thought the kids would fall for it.

I had to laugh.

My seventh-grade-self had been in this pickle once before. On my watch, a neighbor boy's gerbil dropped dead from . . . what? . . . boredom? Sorrow? Migraines induced by my seventies-era daisy wallpaper?

Anyway, I'd attempted that legendarily bad idea of the "switch-eroo." It did not go well. (*"That's* not Brownie!" the kid had howled in despair.)

So when she kindly suggested a replacement fish, I poo-poo'd the scheme.

"Aw, it's just a fish," I said with great level-headedness. "The kids'll be *fine*."

Having read too much lately about "helicopter parents" protecting their progeny from all suffering, I mustered a noble attitude. *I will not shield them from this pain*, I thought. I will walk them through the valley of the shadow of the flushing toilet. And our spines will be stronger for it . . . or some nonsense like that.

Yet for a thousand miles of highway, I dreaded that empty bowl. Because as much as they basically ignored the fish's presence, the kids still prayed for Shiny at night, wrote about him in their school journals, talked about seeing him when we got back home.

The minute we walked in the door, I made a beeline for the bowl in grim expectancy. But there was the fish, tooling around right-side-up.

For two hours of magical thinking, I deluded myself into believing Shiny had made a Lazarus-like recovery. I marveled at his fortitude.

Then I found the note: "Meet Shiny's cousin." I've never been so relieved to have my instructions ignored in all my life.

What a joy to come back home to my own pillow and a mound of laundry—instead of the cold, lifeless corpse of a family friend.

I want to be that kind of neighbor. Someone who hears the voice protesting, "Oh, there's nothing you can do!" or "Don't worry about it, I'll be okay!" and sees it for the lie it is and extends a kindness anyway (be it a casserole, dust rag, or soft shoulder).

We need people who are willing to sidle up alongside us—even when we were all geared up to face the funeral music alone.

I want to be that kind of a friend—the one who shows up in the clutch. Preferably with cookies. And if need be, a fish.

The Story of the Long-Nosed Boy in the Smoldering Shorts

October 2009

It all began with an innocent assignment of show-and-tell, but it ended with my little boy's pants on fire.

And we're not just talking about some smoldering ember either. We're talking five-alarm barn-burner. Britches fully ablaze.

Before I get into the scurrilous details, I must first confess my part in these crimes.

I may have been a *tad* overambitious. This was Will's first real home-work assignment as a kindergartener. And it seemed easy enough. He was to come up with an object starting with "F" and expound upon it ever so briefly in front of the class.

Since he'd just made a plane out of Legos, I suggested in my motherly genius that it would surely pass for a "fighter jet." Thus our ill-fated quest on Wikipedia began, searching for fun facts he could relate about jets breaking the sound barrier (as if I even know what that means twenty years out of high school) and printing pictures of real-life jets (in case the other kids couldn't decipher what his home-made contraption was supposed to be).

I had him fully prepped, briefed, and equipped to knock their tiny collective socks off. As soon as he stepped off the bus, I was pressing him for a full report.

"It was great!" he said. "Even better than I thought it would be!"

As I badgered him for details, he went on to say he'd given some grossly inaccurate figure about how fast fighter jets go. And he made a big show of saying that the teacher put his Lego on display for the rest of the day.

I beamed with pride, patting myself on the back for such excellent parenting.

Until the next afternoon, that is.

That's when I tossed Will a seemingly softball question: "So who did show-and-tell today?"

Will began to explain that since no one had done show-and-tell yesterday . . . and, well, I didn't hear another word out of his mouth.

"Wait. What do you mean *no one* did show-and-tell yesterday?" I quizzed him. "*You* did show-and-tell yesterday, *right?*"

Our minds were both scrambling to come up with the right answer. The right answer, of course, didn't exist. Because the answer was no. *He hadn't done show-and-tell at all.*

The truth was that when the teacher asked kids to share, he'd never even opened his mouth. He'd made the whole thing up. The fun facts, the glorious display, the sunny report on how "it went better than I thought it would." Every word of it . . . lies.

My head started spinning, which caused way too many words to fall out. Words about crushing disappointment and webs of deceit and lying boys getting eaten by wolves.

Lucky for Will, I had to stop the car (and the rant) to get gas. I spent my gas pump time-out breathing deeply, counting to a thousand, and trying to figure out just how to hammer a lesson home without *actually* hammering him.

Maybe the gas fumes were going to my head, but I started thinking about the pressure I'd put on the kid. And I thought about how shy he is. And I thought about how he'd tried so hard not to let me down.

So when I got back in the car, I tried some calmer words. Words about trustworthiness and forgiveness and grace.

And we had a little moment there. Back home, we bonded over Nilla Wafers, and it seemed we had an understanding. My hope was renewed. The slow drumbeat of back-patting began again in earnest.

That's when he headed to the bathroom.

"Did you flush?" I asked upon his return, knowing full well he hadn't.

"Yep," he lied. The kid never even batted an eye.

In an instant, I envisioned teenage Will staggering into the kitchen, spinning yarns about why his breath smelled like a frat house, leading to a splitting headache over my child's moral decline at the ripe old age of five. This thinking led to a whole new slew of words—not all of them so full of grace.

Sigh.

Something tells me this is going to take more than one tidy little "teachable moment."

At this rate, it might just take Robert De Niro and a home polygraph kit.

Planes, Trains, Automobiles, and the Occasional Rickshaw

December 2008

The best laid plans of mice and moms go oft awry. And sometimes they get rammed in the rear.

Picture, if you will, our family of four happily ensconced in our Volvo station wagon. (If you don't know what we look like, might I suggest casting the Jolie-Pitts?)

Like something out of a folksy Thanksgiving song, over the river and through I-95, to Radio City Music Hall we went.

It was Lucy's third birthday, which seemed the perfect time to do something that *seemed* like it was for her, but secretly was for *me*. (She wouldn't remember it anyway.) Seeing the Rockettes kick up their shiny holiday heels was one of those iconic experiences I'd always wanted to check off my list, and this was the big day.

It was about to get way bigger.

So there we were, crossing a busy Connecticut bridge and minding our own happy birthday business, when the first domino fell. Without warning, the car in front of us went from going seventy-five miles an hour to none, skidding to a stop in front of us. Brakes were slammed (even the imaginary one on the passenger side floorboard . . . you know the one), but it was too late. We had nowhere left to go but right into that bumper. Not hard, but enough to put a definite dent in things.

For that one frozen moment, we sat there stunned, not believing our crappy luck. And for that one frozen moment, we forgot there were *other* cars on the road—until one nailed us from behind in a great jarring blow.

That did it. Out of nowhere came air bags, chemical fumes, and cars whizzing by. Faces appeared at the window to see if we were okay. And we were. Everyone was.

Still, I couldn't help crying those dazed, frightened tears. Those tears of "what could have happened." Those tears of "I'm going to miss the freaking Rockettes."

As Bill pulled off the road, I crawled into the backseat and wedged myself between the kids' car seats—all of us rattled, not sure what to say or do next until Will said what we were all thinking. His four-year-old mouth turned down, his eyes welled up, and he sobbed, "But I wanted to see the *showwwww*."

I did the mature thing and sobbed right back, "I did toooo . . ."

Our car was now a leaky metal accordion, dead on the roadside. Its driving days were over. To top things off, there were no cars to rent that Saturday morning; rental car places apparently keep even worse hours than bankers.

Our only wheels now were the tow truck's. And by some miracle, those were enough.

I wouldn't have dreamed an angel could come to earth in a shirt embroidered with the name Wayne, but here's what that saintly tow truck driver did: he dragged our beat-up station wagon with four emotionally beat-up riders inside (diagonally, I might add) down the interstate, across town, and right up to the front door of the nearest train station.

We clamored sideways out of our tow-truck chariot, waved a hearty goodbye to our Good Samaritan, and hopped onto a train—four hobos with air bag debris in their hair riding the rails toward the big city, the fulfillment of a dream, and the happy utilization of some really expensive tickets.

We took six modes of transit that day (take that, Steve Martin!)—station wagon, tow truck, train, subway, taxi, and my personal favorite, rickshaw. (There were *four* of us giggling like criminally insane people in that tiny contraption, but we gave the poor guy a nice tip to help pay for his future visit to the chiropractor.)

By hook or by crook, we managed to stagger from the grim wreckage of our day into the bright lights of Radio City Music Hall.

Even as we settled into our seats in the darkened theater, mesmerized by leggy dancers kicking without care, I couldn't look away from my little girl in the red bow sitting beside me. And I couldn't keep the tears from coming again.

This time, the tears fell not because of what had been lost, but because we didn't miss a thing. Not the show, not the adventure, and not one moment of the precious little life we were celebrating that day.

Anything could have happened. Some of it did. But we had far more to celebrate by the end of that madcap day than at its beginning.

We had made it. We were alive and well and together and sharing something magical—even when common sense said this day (like our car) was a total loss.

Only by God's grace and the gift of human kindness had we made it there. Come to think of it, I'm pretty sure those are the only things that'll get us through the rest of life's misadventures, too.

So let me just say thanks, Wayne, wherever you are. You quite literally saved the day.

You (and that poor, disfigured rickshaw driver) definitely earned your wings.

PART III

GROWING UP (OR IN THAT GENERAL DIRECTION)

I have no stomach for "coming-of-age" movies. Zilch.

If there are cigarettes to be snuck or skirts to be hiked or car windows to be steamed—or if the DVD cover says one word about "blossoming" or "deflowering"—I'm *out*.

Point me toward the Disneys—or even the Scorceses. Just don't make me watch that in-between, teenage-erotic-journey stuff.

Watching a child's innocence fade is just not my favorite. It makes me sad. It makes me fretful. It makes me want to lock my children in the basement without Wi-Fi.

It also prompts me to write a lot of words (as you'll read in this section) about growing up—and how I'd rather just avoid the whole nasty business like a bad coming-of-age movie. But I can't.

I have to face it. I have to embrace it. I have to love my children right through it to the other side—when we can finally get past all this and have a good laugh about pit hair together.

Coming of age, they are. Coming to grips, I must.

That actually sounds like something the wisest and wrinkliest of Jedi Masters would say. He would actually say, "Do, or do not. There is no try."

Shut up, you stupid shriveled California Raisin.

I'm moving as fast as I can here.

Tag Sale Trauma:
My Memory Has Just Been Sold

July 2009

I think I've gone and put a hex on myself.

We just had a yard sale, and I sold all our baby stuff—the strollers, the swing, the tugboat mobile. All of it.

That, of course, can only mean one thing: the stork's on the next flight in. I have brazenly taunted the fertility gods, a dangerous game indeed.

Even worse, I'm finding out how painful all this sloughing off of "baby fat" can be.

Take, for example, the lady at our yard sale who snatched up the precious Mother Goose duvet that had once adorned our baby's crib. She was pleased as punch to tell me she was turning it into a bed for her *cocker spaniel*. (This was heartrending information I did *not* need to know.)

Then a pack of professional tag-salers who didn't speak English worked me over good, making off with a towering pile of my daughter's soft pink things for a measly five bucks.

I know, I know. I ought to be happy that my kids' cast-offs have found new homes.

But standing in that yard, stuffing all my tender baby memories into garbage bags and passing them off to strangers, I felt a new kinship with the J. Geils Band.

My blood ran cold. My memory had just been sold.

In my head, I know this process was good and necessary—both for me *and* our basement. (The hoarding tendency runs strong and deep in my family tree, so this was one small strike against becoming someone who makes a maze to the front door out of old *TV Guides*.)

It was clearly time to part with some stuff.

And, apparently, some of that stuff was ready to part with *me*. After all, time does have a way of loosening our grip on our treasures on earth, where moth and dust and spit-up doth corrupt.

Getting ready for this sale, I pored through box after box of baby clothes with an "awww" on my lips and a familiar tenderness in my heart.

I'd hold up each tiny outfit, preparing to be swept away by lovely Dreft-smelling memories. But onesie by onesie, I was slapped in the face with all these angry mustardy stains, now marring the front of everything soft and sweet that my children ever drooled upon.

I'm the first to admit that I'm not much of a housekeeper, but I *swear* on a stack of Mini Boden catalogs that all of those clothes went in the bin clean.

All I can guess is that somewhere through those years of dank, dark basement living, a lurking blob of yellow corroded like a leaky battery all over my gauzy motherly memories.

Take, for example, the darling outfit my son wore home from the hospital. I would literally lay awake nights fretting over which going-home outfit I'd choose, like I was Sarah Jessica Parker with throngs of paparazzi lying in wait for us outside the hospital doors.

I finally decided (like it *mattered*) on a soft reversible sweater with baby blue on one side, tiny pencil-drawn cows prancing through the air on the other. Today those cows look like they're dodging the steaming piles of Grey Poupon that are somehow *everywhere*.

No amount of OxiClean can save those cows now.

Thankfully, the stain blob didn't get its mitts on everything I'd stowed away, which means I'll keep more of it than I probably should.

I'll definitely hold onto the hospital-issue baby hats topped with curling ribbon, the roll-neck sweater hand-knit by a friend, the his-and-hers smocked Christmas outfits (worn at an age when smocking on a male child was socially acceptable and, in the South, *encouraged*).

I've tucked away these tokens of babyhood in their own special box (okay, *boxes*). Now and then, I'll stumble upon them and have a moment.

But lots more of it had to go, because as much as I'd like to, I can't hold onto everything. It's not healthy. There's no room. And we do have to park our cars someplace.

Even among those things I most desperately want to hold onto in my greedy grip, sometimes the passage of time just doesn't allow it.

Things change.

They fall apart.

They yellow.

They fade.

They grow up.

They move on.

They move out.

(Hold on . . . wait a minute . . . we *are* still talking about the stuff in the basement, right?)

Parenting Without a Net—or a Leash

July 2008

No matter how many gratuitous child-proofing tools I've bought in my parenting life, the sight of a toddler on a leash still weirds me out.

I can't help but feel that these well-meaning parents—in the name of "safety"—have crossed some line that shouldn't be crossed, reducing Little Johnny to the level of family poodle.

Just the other night at a local pizza joint, we watched a toddler checking out with great enthusiasm the restaurant's model trains—all while tethered to dear old dad by a length of bungee cord.

Let me say this once more in case you missed it: the child was looking at *toy trains behind Plexiglass*. He was *not* at the running of the bulls.

I give you the latest victim of Bubble Wrap Parenting.

————————

From the moment the stick turns blue, we're told the world is teeming with pointy/sharp/evil things bent on our child's destruction. We are called upon to arm ourselves to the teeth with safety gadgets—from baby knee pads to wipe warmers to germ-free grocery cart cushions. It's gone a bit off the rails, if you ask me.

I mean, have you seen this contraption called a Bumper Bonnet? The *piéce de résistance* of overkill safety schwag, this tiny styro-helmet is the go-to accessory of the season for your favorite accident-prone toddler to sport around the house. (I cannot stress enough that this thing must always remain *in your house* and *never* appear in public.)

This is all little more than a manufactured fear vortex, designed to separate neurotic new parents from their money and their good sense. But I don't know a new parent over the age of thirty who doesn't get completely sucked into it.

I know. I have a worthless set of infant "sleep positioners" to prove it.

Don't get me wrong. Some of this stuff is truly lifesaving (like that newfangled breathing monitor they've invented for newborns. No joke, a friend's baby is alive today because of it). But mostly, we get caught up in a whirlwind of overthinking and overdoing and overcompensating, buying into whatever might shield our children from every possible hurt and inconvenience. Our focus becomes so fixed on how we can protect and shelter at all costs that we don't even realize: *that's not our job.*

Helping our kids coast through life unscathed has never been the goal of parenting—even if it *was* achievable. Life is full of sharp edges. Kids will run into them.

Helping our children pick themselves up and dust themselves off, ready to take on life's next pointy coffee table—now *that's* the goal.

And that's where I'm trying to find my way now as a mother. I've been so steeped in the overprotective culture of baby care that I am regularly shocked to find my babies growing older and insisting (sometimes with screeching), "I want to do it myself!"

Instead of letting them—which would also mean letting them (and me) experience peril or frustration—I've been too quick to rush in, take over, fix things, and do for them what they could be doing for themselves.

I jerk the shirt over the head, I snatch the toothbrush away and do it "right," I dutifully pick up their messes. I forget that they can—and *must*—learn how to fasten that seat belt, button that shirt, wipe that hind end.

Maybe I don't keep my kids on a leash. But I also don't let them struggle enough, let them try and fail enough, let them do for themselves enough. And by not giving them a chance to fail, I'm not giving them a chance to succeed, either—or to get good enough at doing laundry so that I don't have to do it anymore.

Now *that*, my friends, is a worthy parenting goal.

Out of the Burrow, Onto the Bus
September 2009

I just sent two kids packing on virgin voyages—one to kindergarten, one to preschool. When it comes to big life transitions, this week was *kind of a big deal*.

Even so, there isn't much new I could say about it that hasn't already been said.

Everyone's first day of kindergarten story has the same cast of characters (i.e., wide-eyed child, weepy mom) and all the usual props (i.e., big empty backpack, gleaming new sneaks, soppy Kleenexes). The mixed bag of stressed-out preparations, wild-eyed cheerleading, and nostalgic weepiness—it's all standard fare.

What I hadn't counted on were the *bunnies*.

––––––––––––

Let's go back to exactly one day before our first-day-of-school drama unfolded, and I'll give you the whole spiel.

So there I was, making some ridiculous bus-shaped cake (which tells you how much I was overthinking all this) when my husband came bounding into the house, yelling and hollering to come outside.

Heavens to Betsy, the man had nearly run over a whole mess of baby bunnies with the lawnmower.

Okay, calm down, everybody. I said "nearly."

Let me state for the record: *no bunnies were harmed in the making of this story*. The blades weren't able to reach through the depths of that tall, willowing grass and the dandelion groves to do any real damage. (Still, those bunnies will *definitely* need counseling.)

Bunny babies had tunneled through the grass in every direction like Bugs Bunny blazing a trail to Albuquerque. There was no nest I could see, no mom to be found. They all just hunkered deep down in random spots all over our front yard.

And there they stayed throughout the night and into the next day. They never moved a tiny muscle. Yet the dandelions grew ever taller, taunting my husband, making him antsy to mow.

What with a kindergartener to get on the bus and salty tears to cry, I was kind of busy that next morning, but I came home from the bus stop with a pocketful of snot rags, a yard full of bunnies, and no clue what I should do.

Was Mama Cottontail coming back? Or had she taken up with a no-account townie rabbit? Should I just let things unfold as nature intended? Or should I assume that nature's intentions are evil and get these sweet babies to safety?

So I researched the matter extensively, which means I read Wikipedia and made a few calls. I found a nice wildlife rehabilitator who said she'd take the bunnies back to her farm where they could frolic and grow old together. That sounded like a far better option than our death-blade yard, so I decided to go with that.

I set to work, scooping up the babies one by one and nestling them into a shoebox lined with a golf towel.

The first bunny barely flinched when set upon by this fifty-foot woman, but the others made me work for it, screeching and flailing and trying to dial 911.

(I literally made baby bunnies *scream*. I do not recommend it.)

Even after they'd been stowed safely inside the box, this bunch did not go calmly into the night. No, the bunnies continued to fling themselves against the lid like popcorn kernels in a JiffyPop bag, which made me hate myself exceedingly and question every decent motive I've ever had.

I mean, maybe the bunny mom had it handled, maybe I was messing with things I shouldn't, or maybe causing a boxful of baby bunnies to stroke out wasn't my best plan. *Maybe.*

All I knew for sure was that I was *trying* with great desperation and big-hearted love to do the right thing—even if I couldn't know for sure what that was.

In a moment of "quiet" reflection (holding a thumping box of frenzied baby bunnies in my lap), it seemed to me that *all* the little creatures around here—in this box *and* in our house—were being wrested from their nests and shoved into places they weren't quite sure about.

Some went with quiet calm, some with an urge to screech and dart back to the hole. Either way, it's been generally uncomfortable and scary for all parties involved.

All the while, there's been this tall crazy lady in the picture—lurching around blindly and stupidly, not quite sure what she's doing, worrying about what happens to the babies without her, worrying about what happens to them if she gets everything all wrong.

But the bunnies had already survived the blades and the box, so I'm hoping that was the worst of it.

I like to picture them now all grown up, scampering in a meadow somewhere, maybe wearing overalls and painting Easter eggs. I have big dreams for those bunnies.

As for my own babies, well, I'm holding out lots of hope for them too . . . hope for all the good things that can happen in their grown-up lives if somehow, some way, despite all the desperate flailing and failings of the fifty-foot woman, we manage to get it right.

Yep, I have big dreams for my babies, too.

Oddly enough, none of them include overalls.

B is for Bird
June 2010

Will just gave me the finger.

Actually, he just (as sweetly as you please) held up his tiny hand and folded each finger down—until only one was left standing. Then he asked with wide-eyed bewilderment, "Mommy, what does this mean?"

The air went out of the room for a minute.

The child is in kindergarten, for crying out loud. He can't even spell his last name (and probably won't till he's twelve). Yet here we are, learning all about the wonderful world of obscene finger gestures. I should never have let him leave the house.

I frankly don't remember much of what I said . . . some mumbo jumbo about it being something hateful that people do . . . something about never, ever doing it.

But I had questions, too, like where the heck did he see this? At circle time, reading *If You Give a Pig a Pancake?*

As best I can gather from Will's recounting of the day's events, his class was doing something math-ish, and Will was counting down the old-fashioned way—on his fingers. Then wham-o, he's down to one. The Big One.

A classmate who's clearly watched too much cable went bananas and raised a giant tattle-taling stink all over this poor, clueless little boy. A boy who'd heretofore looked at his middle finger and saw only the number one with a hangnail. A boy who was now sobbing into my lap, thinking he'd done something awful he didn't even know was awful. A boy who was convinced the other kids didn't like him because they were trying to get him into trouble. A boy who now knew the meaning of an ugly gesture I'd hoped wouldn't show up until . . . I don't know . . . *never?*

I was watching the first cracks form in my child's sweet protective shell of innocence.

I hate this part.

I hate worrying about what kids are doing and saying on the bus away from my watchful eye. I hate hearing about kids "sexting" or watching porn on their tablets or wearing microscopic scraps of denim they laughingly call "skirts."

It seems like everything in our culture is sinking to new (and ever earlier) lows of skankiness.

This is where parenting starts to feel like driving on black ice. We know there's nasty stuff out there, but we coast along blithely until—out of nowhere—the skidding takes us by surprise. Then we spin off together, sweating and gripping the wheel and clamoring for a way to gain some traction in our children's lives.

Talking about bird-flipping with a six-year-old—that'll do wonders for reminding you that this gig is about more than giving them rides or improving their T-ball swing. Infinitely more.

Ready or not, my husband and I have been given the never-a-day-off job of prepping the road under four little feet—in the hope that when our kids hit those slippery patches, we've given them something solid to grip onto.

But I'm with Carrie Underwood on this one. I've had this one heartbreaking conversation and already I'm throwing my hands over my eyes and begging Jesus to take the wheel.

Really, that's the best idea I've heard yet.

The Tooth Fairy Haters Club
June 2011

Lucy's bottom tooth can do this really cool, nauseating trick. It can fold all the way down at a full ninety-degree angle and still *not fall out*. And by golly, Lucy intends to keep it that way. Right where it sits. No matter what this may mean for her summer corn-on-the-cob eating.

When it comes to losing her first tooth, my girl is as unhinged as that incisor.

From the moment she felt that first wiggle, she started mourning the loss ("I don't want to lose a part of me!"), rationalizing that five-year-olds aren't old enough for tooth-shedding ("But I still suck my fumb!") and launching personal attacks against that low-down, snake-in-the-grass Tooth Fairy ("I *hate* the Toof Fairy! I don't want her to eat my toof!").

For Lucy, no amount of cash payment under the pillow is a fair trade for this treasured part of her young life.

Come to think of it, I'm in no rush for that tooth to go, either. What good can come of this? *Puberty*? I think not.

But it's not just the tooth. I'm noticing my baby girl has actual calf muscles now. No more soft rubber-band wrists. No more chubby thigh creases. Just the slender beginnings of muscle.

Even worse, she sometimes has the nerve to ask me, like a true tween-to-be, "Mom, can you leave the room? I was doing something."

I know, she's not kicking me out to finish up her cigarette; she's probably just planning another surprise party for her matching giraffe loveys, Gigi and Emily.

Still, I'm witnessing my girl easing her way up the growth chart in all these nearly undetectable little ways—each change adding up to someone new. Those are the times I put on a crazy-eyed smile and start fumbling for the imaginary brake cord dangling over my head.

A friend of mine has a daughter just about to turn twelve. She told me once with genuine surprise, "All these years I looked at my friends with teenagers, and I never thought it'd *actually* happen to me."

My mom brain cons me into thinking that every phase is a permanent condition . . . as though my daughter will always say words wrong in that cutesy little kid way, as though she'll always wobble along on training wheels, as though she'll always be right here hiding behind my leg. She won't.

Change comes. Teeth fall out. Teeth grow back in as bucky Chiclets to ruin the first-grade picture, only to get plastered with shiny teenage braces. (Years from now, they'll fall out again, only to be replaced with gleaming new ones floating in a glass of Efferdent.)

Yes, change comes. But surely change isn't always something to be feared.

I spend a lot of time watching my daughter zipping like a fiend on her Barbie scooter, her thick blonde tresses in a furry blaze behind her.

And I remember how—not so long ago—a walk around this block took hours. Every fallen acorn was of infinite interest, and great mounds of them had to be deposited one-by-one into a drainage grate.

From this same post, I now watch the body in motion of my little girl, embracing life with great full-speed-aheadness. And it is exhilarating.

There's a twinge of nostalgia for the days of acorn gathering. But mostly, it's a joy to watch this girl on the verge.

Still my baby. But not for long.

The Leaning Tower of Binders (and Other Wonders of the Middle-School World)

August 2014

I have a boy just starting middle school, so out of nowhere, my main concern in all of life has become *binders*.

From the moment I got the school supply list in the mail, I have been slavish to its every whim. I filled the cart with notebooks (spiral and non), packs of new pencils (colored and non—though we have a forest of them already), and a huge towering stack of binders.

In case you're out of the school loop, these ringed wonders have replaced the relics we once knew as *books*. They are also the black holes into which a boy's daily shuffle of papers are sucked and never heard from again.

Let me assure you—there is a zero-percent chance of all those gargantuan, pointy notebooks fitting into my ten-year-old's backpack— at least on the days he wants to eat.

The lunchbox clearly has to go.

This leads me to the totally logical conclusion that I've screwed this up somehow. Maybe I didn't get the *right* binders.

I have become obsessed with binder perfection—for them to all fit just right, for the corners not to be too sharp or the cover too lame, for the weight not to stoop Will's bird-like shoulders and doom him to a back-braced adolescence.

I want everything to be perfect—the binders, his middle school experience, his entire existence on planet Earth. (I acknowledge that this may not be reasonable.)

Bigger issues may be at work under this shiny Trapper Keeper surface—like how I know (and he doesn't yet) that middle school is hard, and I'm scared for him.

Kindergarten was supposed to be the ultimate childhood transition, and it's definitely big. But it's also the sweetest, cuddliest teddy bear of a place to send one's beloved babies.

Middle school is a different animal—a much gnarlier one. I vividly remember it sucking. I remember looking the dorkiest I've ever looked. I remember sticking out and not being cool and doing things all gangly and wrong.

So if I could *just* get the binders right for him, maybe all of this humiliation could be avoided.

That's how a mom thinks, anyway.

We know it doesn't really work that way. Somewhere inside, we know.

But still we try to fix the things we can by sending our children off with the right stuff, or the cutest back-to-school ensemble, or something (anything) that says Under Armour on it. All the rest of it is utterly and miserably beyond our control.

Most of it's even beyond our knowing about (like when you have a male child whose standard answer is "nothing" to the "What'd you do today" question.)

So my kid will come home from middle school each day, and I will ask about his day. He won't tell me a fat lot. I will then dig through that towering pile of binders and search for clues. This is a wild new journey we're embarking on—him with ten pounds of supplies strapped to his wee back, me with shoulders heaped with motherly concern watching him go.

What I am sending him off with may not be perfect, it may not fit quite right, and it may not be the coolest ever.

But all the love and prayers I've crammed into every square inch ought to count for something . . . maybe almost everything.

Still, I did keep the receipt on those binders.

Just in case.

Dear Elementary School:
A Breakup Letter
June 2015

Dear Elementary School, I wish I knew how to quit you.

My baby girl's last day to walk your dear, sweet, rainbow-hued halls is today. I am not handling it well.

In fact, I couldn't face seeing you today. I'm a weepy puffy-eyed mess, reminiscent of Tammy Faye Bakker at full boil—just without the mascara. (I didn't even bother with makeup today. I knew it wouldn't last.)

My youngest child is being shoved from your cozy, construction paper–lined nest and forced to fly to middle school next year. We'd give anything to linger at least one more year in your loving arms, but we must soldier on—and away from you. Which kind of blows.

But before we go, I had to tell you how I feel.

I will miss you dearly, Elementary School.

I will miss your Technicolor playgrounds filled with sparkly sneakers stretching from your swing sets to the sky. As far as I can tell, the big kids have fields and basketball courts and a lot of loitering.

I will miss the little kids walking your halls single-file. There may be imps who dawdle and goof and do the occasional cartwheel, but there are no marauding bands of tweens here. I like that.

I will miss your bulletin boards with the bubble letters, the teachers' smiley stickers on homework papers, and your miles and miles of lamination.

I will miss your miniature desks, and your miniature chairs, and your miniature water fountains that will one day seem like a scene out of Munchkin Land to my all-grown-up kids.

I will miss your teachers. They have helped me raise my children so thoughtfully, so skillfully, so generously; I truly consider them friends now. (I mean, I barely know my older middle schooler's teachers' names. It's just different now.)

I will miss your never-ending cavalcade of plays, concerts, and assemblies. I won't lie to you; they were *long*. Half the time, we couldn't hear what anyone was saying. And those screechy renditions of *Hot Cross Buns* on the recorder might have caused permanent hearing loss. But those were big days for our kids, and they gave us parents a chance to take pictures of our kids in paper antlers and sniffle our way through the school song. I'll miss that stuff. *Most* of it.

I will miss your bins of busted-up crayons and crusty glue sticks. You always had tools at the ready when inspiration struck and stick figures were begging to be drawn.

I will miss your little-kid artwork all over the walls. Middle-school art gets a little moody and crying-clownish. I like your happy handprints.

Bear with me. I'm getting a little sappy and morose. I get like that at the big moments—and this one feels huge to me.

My head tells me it's time to move on, and I know eventually I will.

It won't take long (less than three months, in fact) before you'll start seeing other people (lots of them). And in time, I'll start to forget you, what you were like, and the moments we shared together.

But, Elementary School, I'll never forget we had something really special for a while.

I know this much is true . . . I could never love another school the way I loved you.

Forever yours,
DeeDee

Birds, Bees, and (for Lack of a Better Word) Coconuts

May 2015

My little boy is getting the sex talk at school today. Somebody get over here and *hold me.*

As Will embarks on the fifth-grade science unit about "human growth and development," the light will dawn on all those weird words I was never enlightened enough to teach him.

I'm sorry, but most of those words are gross (except for vas deferens, which sounds kind of fancy.) I much prefer the vagaries of "down there."

Today, he will watch that video (if he ever gets out from under his desk) with drawings of girls and boys "developing," which boils down to getting hairy and growing "coconuts." (That's Will's word. I swear I didn't teach him that one.)

Today, the shales will fall off his eyes, and he will become acquainted with "sanitary napkins."

Today, my child will learn where babies come from, without any mention of storks or cabbage patches or God's eternal mystery.

Today is the end of the innocence.

———————

I *know*, I'm painfully repressed. I own that. But allow me to play for you the full-length, unedited director's cut of my mother telling me all about the birds and the bees.

Mom: There's some stuff under the sink when you need it. ("Stuff" = Kotex.)

Me: Um, okay.

The End.

Good talk.

This is the same woman who anonymously left a box of KY Jelly wrapped in a paper towel on my nightstand on my wedding day. So yeah, I come by it honest.

But because so painfully little was said at my house, I *know* that it's needed. And I do want things to be different with my own kids so that Mom and Dad are safe places to go to with their fears, questions, and gross words (though my male child is unlikely to ever speak of these things again).

I get it. I really do.

I'm just not quite ready for all that to be said *today*. I can't remotely get a handle on how we got here this quick.

But ready or not, we're here.

So today it's time for game face, for bear hugs for the traumatized kid about to walk through my door, for all the elevating words I can muster about "God's design," and for a healthy dose of silliness and conspiratorial laughter (because seriously y'all, it *is* funny).

It's time to face the music and be the mom I want to be—not some mute, distant shadow mom out of a John Hughes movie, but one who's there, who gets it, who knows all the words and isn't afraid to use them (if there is *absolutely no other choice*).

It's time to show my kid a mom who loves him desperately—in spite of all his weird hairiness to come.

Evicting the Thirteen-Year-Old Inside (and Other Life Goals)

September 2015

A coworker grabbed me as I walked into work the other day and announced, "Hey! There's a picture in the paper today of a woman who looks *just like you!*"

In a flash, he was gone to retrieve it, leaving me to wonder: What great beauty could this be? Julia Roberts, perhaps? Jennifer Lawrence? Ms. Hathaway from *The Beverly Hillbillies?*

At that moment, he plunks down before me a picture of a *man.*

This man was dressed as a woman (quite nicely, I should add), which is what I tried to impress upon my colleague in a distressed voice much too loud for an office setting.

"This is Eddie Redmayne," I insisted, searching his eyes for any clues of irony or taunting. "A male actor. Playing a *transgender woman.*" (Uncomfortably long pause.) "You're saying I look like a *man.*"

He didn't believe me until he read the caption, so I honestly don't think he was trying to kill my soul.

Still, if you're going to make a big hairy deal about *how I look just like someone*, could you at least cheer me up and make it a *female* someone?

———

The next day I had a mammogram, which was the worst.

Sitting in the waiting robe in a flimsy robe, waiting to get naked in front of a stranger, I made the mistake of forgoing *Family Circle* and flipping through a *Vanity Fair* centerfold on Sofia Vergara. She is one of the few people on Earth whose birthday suit is her best look.

Let's just say, this exercise was in no way helpful.

Sofia Vergara must have to block out *hours* for her mammogram, there's so much ground to cover. I'm pretty sure that the cute little technician took one look at me *sans* gown and thought, "I sure hope we can find something under there to scan."

Body image is a bitch. And as much as I've grown up and into myself in some lovely, healthy ways, those old insecurities of the stoop-shouldered thirteen-year-old inside never really die.

I'm not consumed with *Seventeen* magazine like I once was, analyzing Jennifer Connelly from the top of her scrunchie to the soles of her high-top Reeboks. By the ripe old age of forty-four, I've accumulated too many other things to worry about, which is just as it should be.

But the thirteen-year-old inside still wants to stuff her bra with tube socks.

The thirteen-year-old inside still sucks in her gut all day—or hides her muffin top under billowing folds of fabric like Stevie Nicks.

Like everybody else, I'm bothered more than I should be about what people think of me and my spider veins and my unruly hair with the grays sticking out and my frumpy wardrobe and my lumpy knees and my pores and my paunch.

I don't care enough to actually do sit-ups (let's not get carried away), but still, I fret.

Still, that thirteen-year-old is there.

The thirteen-year-old inside especially likes to pop out whenever my little girl takes my picture. (Lucy's low to the ground so she always gets me at the worst possible angles.)

"Oh, delete that! I look a fright!" I always screech, which is exactly what you should *never* say to a child who's taking her mother's cues along the path to a healthy self-esteem.

Without fail, Lucy will say something sweet back to me like, "Why do you always say that? You're beautiful!"

And, it's true.

Perhaps it's not "beauty" as the world sees beauty, not like a starlet cinching her boobs together, getting ready for her close-up.

But to my daughter, I'm beautiful. And I feel exactly the same way about her.

When I look at my baby girl, I am overcome. She's perfect to me. I could eat up every bit of her.

My Maker feels the same way about me—yet in infinitely deeper and wider and more unfathomable ways. My physical imperfections are meaningless to Him, except those lines and scars that made me who I am. Those He loves. (He showed off His own hard-earned scars as beauty marks, so I know.)

I'm invaluable and beautiful and precious in His sight. He says so.

Even when the robe is off and my every flaw is exposed, I must cling to that. It's really all that matters.

And even when the other fifth-graders at the party are taking selfies of their "six-packs" (yeah, that happened), I pray that Lucy will cling to what's true. That she'll tell me about it later while grabbing her belly and exclaiming, "I love my chub!" (That happened, too.) That she will see beauty as something more, something deeper, something the mean girls can't dig their claws into, something eternal.

I want richer, sweeter, wiser, cooler, lovelier things for the both of us.

Because here's the deal: I may never be fully rid of you, but I'm kind of over you, thirteen-year-old self.

You're *so* 1984.

PART IV

FEATS OF STRENGTH

Dear Reader, this is one of the shortest sections in the whole book. That's because it's about "sports and activities."

Except for my studly husband, our family does not excel at sports and activities. In fact, we generally refrain from sports and activities. And when we *do* participate in sports and activities, our athletic performance is almost always (how shall I put this delicately?) *undistinguished*.

If you have ever cringed and ducked at the incoming flight of a Wiffle ball, if you've ever logged *zero-point-zero* seconds in the flexed arm hang during a presidential fitness test, if you have never imbibed a protein shake on purpose, this section is for you.

But, my sporty friends, don't lose heart. Oh, do read on.

I have to believe that even families brimming with Adonis-like humanoids have their own hidden insecurities under all those rippling muscles. Maybe somewhere deep down within that aerobically supercharged body of yours, you can even relate to our suffering. Or laugh at it.

Either way, I'll never know. That's the beauty of it.

P.S. I'm sure my son would want you to know that, after years of exploring the various sports and activities discussed in this section, he has at long last discovered cross-country running. He even goes so far as to call it "his thing."

Just when all hope was lost, are those the distant strains of *"We Will Rock You"* I hear? Cue up the Jumbotron, y'all.

Cheering on the Boy
with the Swiss Cheese Mitt

March 2011

Our first-grader is officially a T-ball graduate. We have now entered The Big Leagues. I am afraid.

Little-kid baseball should be harmless enough, right? All the kid has to do is upgrade from hitting off a stick to hitting in midair, right?

But here's the rub: It's *fine* to stink at T-ball. It's even expected.

It's fine to pick those daisies (or your nose).

It's fine to never even *see* that ball skidding between your legs.

The grown-ups at a T-ball game will all throw up their hands and squeal with delight. "Isn't that adorable?" they hoot.

But that's *T-ball*, y'all.

Once you upgrade to *real* baseball, that's when the laughter stops. Antics that used to be cute aren't so cute anymore, and that weak amateur-hour stuff starts getting called by its real name—"sucking."

So here we are, about to send our hapless little boy onto that field, still stuck in his T-ball time warp—still sucking, still daisy-picking—while I'm betting all the other kids have spent their entire winter drilling steroids and dragging logs through the tundra like it's *Rocky IV*.

(I didn't say these were *rational* fears . . .)

Sometimes I'd give anything for our kids to be jocks. Man, it'd make life so much easier.

I could cozy up on the sidelines with all the other jock moms, commiserating about our rough-and-tumble boys who live to play with a ball all day every day (instead of quizzing myself in shamed silence, "When's the last time my kid actually threw a ball?").

I could cheer lustily over our little champion, instead of wincing, rolling my eyes, or hiding under the bleachers while another ball falls through the gaping hole in my child's mitt.

I could dream of a free ride to college on the wings of golden Nikes. It'd just be nice, that's all I'm saying.

But even as I write those words, I have to wonder if maybe—just *maybe*—those jock parents wish their kids were something else, too, something they imagine would make their lives or their children's lives better somehow.

Maybe they wish their kids were book-smart enough to zip through all forty-five *Magic Tree House* books, or that they could draw something other than a dead-eyed stick figure, or that they'd just once touch that guitar Santa brought them for Christmas.

There's always *something*.

At our house, we wish Will showed even the faintest interest in kicking, throwing, hitting, dribbling, or catching a spherical object. We'd settle for just *one* of the five.

But what do I have to complain about? Will's a sweet, happy, healthy kid. He likes school, he's a mean Lego builder; he loves birds, animals, and his little sister. He's got his own thing going, and at the risk of sounding like a self-esteem poster, that's okay, too.

The truth is, I could stand to spend a little more time loving who our son is and a lot less time lamenting what he's not.

Besides, he's just turned seven. It's hardly time to give up and doom him to a life in the basement playing Dungeons & Dragons.

Who knows? Maybe he'll love baseball and being part of the team. Maybe through this experience, he'll tap into his inner Sporty Spice. *Maybe.*

Or maybe he'll end up being less athlete than Mathlete.

Whatever. Doesn't matter.

I've got my big foam finger ready. Either way, that kid will be someone worth cheering about.

First Position's Last Stand
September 2010–February 2011

I talk to a lot of mothers in my mom-centric world, and I'm starting to worry I might be the only one obsessed with this.

Ever since the day five years ago when a pixilated space alien on the screen was pronounced to be our unborn baby girl, I started carrying around a picture of her in my head.

I'm pretty sure that picture was unduly influenced by minivan commercials—like the one where the door slides open and a puppy pile of pink, pint-sized ballerinas tumbles out.

Blonde bun, pudgy leotard belly, shimmery tutu—that, to me, is the quintessential look of little girl-ness. And ever since ever, I've longed for the day I could put my Lucy in that picture—whether the girl cared a lick about it or not.

This might be a sickness.

———————

A year and a half ago, I rushed to sign Lucy up for a tiny tot ballet class in town, the one with the lovely old British lady who played the piano by the barre. My heart hurt just thinking of all that pastel preciousness; I had a whole color palette of leotards ready to go.

But days before Lucy's first class, I got the call. The lovely old British lady was retiring. The studio was closing; my dream was shattering. (Okay, that's a tad melodramatic, but it did bum me out.)

One year later, I signed Lucy up for yet another ballet program, one gracious enough to let Lucy (still uninspired by multiple viewings of *Angelina Ballerina*) take a couple of trial lessons first.

Because maybe you've noticed, I'm using first-person possessives like "*my* dream" a lot. The sad truth is that Lucy has about 0.00001 percent interest in this. I'm trying to figure out if that makes me some kind of overbearing stage mother. (Don't answer that.)

But I also know my children. They're not the "me first" types, clamoring to try new stuff. They're more of the "we're not so sure about this, can't we just stay at home?" types. My kids need a nudge, if not a full-on shove with a very large and pointy-toed shoe.

I know them, *and* I know *me*. I never took the first dance lesson, but all my friends had those huge photo collages of themselves from tap and jazz class, bedecked in sequins from the tops of their feathery fedoras to the bottoms of their patent leather tap shoes.

While I don't remember ever wanting to be in that picture (or the flapper dress), I do remember the stoop-shouldered shame of being the gangliest oaf ever dragged onto a dance floor. (Just picture weird flailing elbows *everywhere*.)

I figured Lucy could use a little oaf-resistance training. It couldn't hurt, and she might shock us all by actually liking it. So I decided to force the ballet issue—despite her protests that she only likes to do "fun dancing" at home.

And even if Lucy never made it past lesson two, at least I'd have that priceless picture from lesson one—my little girl in a leotard and bun, living out her mother's dream.

If only for one afternoon.

Ballet lessons dragged on for five more months—though I probably should have put us all out of our misery after two freebies and the cute photo.

Every week, I'd wedge Lucy's love handles into that powder blue sausage casing, fantasizing that *this* would be the week that launched her love affair with tutus. And every week, she'd flop around in there, doing whatever it is they do behind closed studio doors. She'd come out smiling, with no visible signs of trauma. But as soon as I'd start cramming her toes into those pink shoes for the next week's class, she'd wail: "But you said I only had to go two tiiiimes!"

Okay, I did sort of say that. We moms say a lot of things we don't mean.

But because she'd survived those first two lessons without a scene (my weird litmus test for success) and because I'd already sprung for all that pricey gear, we forged ahead.

Well, more like *I* forged ahead and dragged Lucy along behind.

I guess I knew deep-down but wasn't ready to admit: Lucy and ballet did not a love connection make.

It's not so bad if ballet's not her thing, thought my rational self. *Something else will be her thing.*

Like lying around the house aimlessly, for example.

Shut up, you weak, pathetic, undisciplined sap! my inner Tiger Mother snapped. *How else do you expect this child to learn the time-honored principles of stick-to-it-iveness, self-discipline, and being able to plié without falling over?*

My inner mothers were at it again.

––––––––––

Then came Lucy's last class of the semester . . . actually, her last class *ever*.

Parents got to watch this time, so I came prepared like a one-man film crew from the six o'clock news, ready to document every angle of first position's last stand. My misty eyes may have been fogging up the lens, but what I saw changed things for me.

In a room full of dainty sprites that looked like they'd pirouetted straight out of a music box, I saw a girl a head taller than the rest.

Where other girls had leotards that gapped around their toothpick legs, Lucy pleasantly filled her elastic to capacity.

Where other girls pointed toes and twirled like they'd been posing in front of a mirror all of their short lives, my dear Lucy affably lumbered.

In a sea of pink tulle, she was Waldo in stripes. One of these was not like the others. And in that moment, I knew. I knew that it was okay to let it go.

There's something else out there for my daughter, but this wasn't it. And we've got lots of time to figure out what that "something else" is.

Lucy's little life is a hall lined with doors to choose. Some will be right, some wrong, some we'll regret never opening, and some we'll wonder if we closed too soon.

Some will open up to the winning car. Some will send her home with his-and-her track suits.

It's a crapshoot. And when it comes to helping our kids find their niche in this life, I wish I had even a smidgen of Kenny Rogers's confidence.

The Gambler. Now *there's* a man who knew when to hold 'em and knew when to fold 'em, knew when to walk away and knew when to run. I'm never quite sure when to do *any of that*.

So the best I can do is keep easing down this hall of doors, trusting my gut, and praying all the way for the wisdom of Solomon. Or if that's too high a mark, God, I'd be fine with the wisdom of Kenny Rogers.

That's pretty good, too.

Our Own Personal Miracle on Ice

February 2012

I saw my old roller skates on a Gymboree poster last week.

The gleaming white leather, the red and blue racing stripes, that chunky red stopper—I'd know those beauties anywhere. And there they were, in all their 1980s glory, on a little girl thirty-five years my junior.

The poster child looked soft and sweet and far less susceptible to full-body casts than the now-forty-year-old who once rolled down hills in them.

I loved those skates. I loved playing "Sonic drive-in" in our driveway, rolling up to the station wagon windows and delivering imaginary vanilla Cokes. I loved my Saturdays at Skateland, where a film of pizza grease glazed the floors by the Donkey Kong machine.

Deep down, I've always wanted my kids to like skating, too. Or at the very least, for the sake of future skating parties, I've wanted my children to rise above the ranks of the desperate wall-clinger or staggering flailer (the one who sends all passersby to the emergency room). Remaining upright and on a forward trajectory 75 percent of the time seems a reasonable skating goal for life.

Besides all that, Will and Lucy are (sigh . . .) native New Englanders. And while this Southern gal wouldn't touch one big toe to a frozen body of water, skating on ponds is what y'all do. So when in Northern Rome, you do as the Northerners do and learn to skate—preferably on actual ice and not pavement, like a sissy.

With two ice skating lessons under my kids' belts, I'm shocked to report—it hasn't been a disaster.

It got off to a wobbly start, as these things do. First of all, I forgot that ice rinks are, well, *freezing*.

What was obvious to hearty New England parents—like how to cover their snow babies in gloves and snow pants and bike helmets (!)—wasn't quite so obvious to me. My underdressed, hatless children were like little lost sheep—shivering, shorn, and being thrown to the ice wolves.

Then there was the sorting of all those sharp-shoed tots into groups.

On that very first day, I heard my daughter's instructor call out, "Lucy, you're over here!" and I did a double take. The disembodied voice seemed to emanate from some chick with a clipboard *way* down at the other end of the rink. I had to squint for a better view.

If she hadn't been so ridiculously far away, I would have jerked that smug Oksana Baiul–wannabe by the ponytail and said, "*Are you kidding me right now? If my daughter knew how to get there, we wouldn't be here.*"

(Okay, I would never have done that, but if she'd been closer, she definitely would have heard me huff in displeasure. *That'd* show her.)

Lucy shot me a quick look of terror and started on her way, baby-stepping a wobbly path to the far reaches of Outer Mongolia. God bless her, banana slugs could've gotten there quicker.

I have to say, watching all this from the sidelines has been downright hilarious. Every session is like a sitcom—complete with a parental laugh track of "whoops" and "whoa Nellies." If the highest form of comedy is the pratfall, then watching these kids stagger and flop makes for forty-five minutes of pure comic gold.

But I wasn't laughing when my surprisingly upright son came off the ice after that first lesson, jumping up and down on his blades, exulting, "I didn't fall that much!"

I wasn't laughing; I was too busy high-fiving.

And I wasn't laughing when Lucy, out of nowhere in lesson two, started hurtling fast across the ice like a girl possessed, slamming into the wall with a giant grin. I wasn't laughing; my mouth was too busy hanging open.

"Jesus must have accepted my prayer," she said on the ride home. "While I was out there, I prayed I wouldn't be the slowest anymore."

You can have your Stanley Cups, your 1980 Team USA wins.

They're a big deal and all, but in a houseful of distinctly non-Olympians, *not* being the slowest . . . *not* falling too much . . . that's what we like to call victory.

That, my friends, is our own personal miracle on ice.

Soccer—*Sanford and Son* Style
June 2013

I sometimes wonder what our back-window stick figure family would look like if we owned a minivan.

Dad with furrowed eyebrows and a power drill?

Mom with exhausted X's for eyes?

Two sun-shunning children with fangs and widow's peaks?

I guarantee you that a happy bouncing ball would be nowhere in sight. I say this with equal parts sadness and smugness: a life lived in folding chairs from the sidelines has not been ours. That is, until Lucy decided she honestly, truly, weirdly wanted to play soccer. I'm talking third-grade, serious-business soccer—where you have to do hard-core stuff like *try out for teams* and *travel to games* (like half an hour away!) and *practice three times a week*.

These kids are so little; I think it's all bonkers—especially if yours is the player who's devoted her entire "soccer career" to the position of head skylarker/daisy picker/ball dodger.

So for months ahead of time, I've been asking this child the same question:

Me: "You're *sure* you want to play soccer next year?"

Lucy, with a nonchalant shoulder shrug: "Sure."

Me: "Really?! You'll have to actually practice and stuff. It's not just for Saturdays anymore ..."

Lucy, another shoulder shrug: "Okay."

Hence, it is with this level of shirt-ripping soccer enthusiasm that we arrived at the big fat official soccer evaluations.

We'd practiced hard for that fateful day (and by "practicing hard," I mean that I'd posted the skills tests on our bulletin board and never looked at it again). We did try to practice—once—using a laundry basket as a goal and a ball that dented when you kicked it.

So yeah, from the moment we arrived at try-outs, it was pretty clear the girl was outmanned. For starters, mine was the only kid there in dingy pink tennis shoes and completely unguarded shins.

One coach all but patted me on the head and said, "You'll want to buy some cleats for her to play in." I mumbled something about out-growing them, hid my face, and shuffled to the next humiliation station.

What I hadn't grasped—as someone who typically avoids this type of thing—was that tonight was all about looking the part. It was about "game face."

We were surrounded by people whose ball never, ever lacked proper inflation, who wore Umbros in their sleep, who got their kids coaching tutors for the off-season, who actually *cared*.

Please know that I say this with all love and adoration, but Lucy's soccer try-out was straight-up *Sanford and Son*.

It was this harum-scarum mash-up of not quite knowing what she was doing or why she was doing it (and doing it in those frowned-upon shoes). Yet she took her naked little shins and all the courage she could muster and ran and kicked and whiffed and tried as best she knew how.

If it were me—and all those grown-ups with stopwatches and clip-boards were studying my sloppy, desperate seven-year-old frame in action—I'd have prayed for that preternaturally green grass to swallow me whole. I would have been scared to death. I would never have gone through with it.

Come to think of it, I never did go out for a team or audition for a play or put myself out there in any way where failure was a possibility. And that's the ultimate whiff—never even trying.

So I'm proud of our brave little ball-dodging Hobo Joe. There could be a soccer ball sticker in our back window's future yet.

But the good money is on those two X'd-out mom eyes. Those, my friend, are a given.

A Bug's Life
(and Slow, Inevitable Death)
June 2010

Author's Note: This is my book, so I'm counting bug-collecting as a "sport." It's outside. Whatevs.

Only one thing gets slug slime off your hands, or so I'm told. Not Wet Wipes or 409 or a Mr. Clean Magic Eraser. Just plain ol' paper towels.

Why, you may ask, do I know this?

Because critter enthusiast Lucy lives here—my fearless explorer of all things creepy, crawly, and equipped with more legs than I am humanly comfortable with.

Having been raised in the South where cockroaches are big enough to saddle and ride, I am no fan of bugs.

The other night (by way of testimony), I screamed from some primal place within me when oncoming headlights revealed a smallish brown spider on my driver's side window. On the *inside*. (It was like one of those B-movies where the babysitter, usually Jennifer Love Hewitt, figures out the murderer is calling from the laundry room. Cue blood-curdling screams and/or delicate fainting.)

With my blood pressure shooting up to stroke levels, I screeched into a bait-and-tackle shop parking lot and launched from the vehicle. It was dark, and the deadly brown recluse (as I imagined it to be) was a good hider, so I drove home with the interior lights ablaze in wide-eyed itchy terror.

Trust me, if a bug so much as steps one spindly leg inside the inner sanctum of our home, I will swoop down on him with a whole arsenal of weapons—be it fistfuls of Kleenex, steel-toed shoes, or a ten-pound September issue of *Vogue*.

I hate bugs and worms and all their hair-raising kin, but my Lucy loves them—to death.

To God's smallest creatures, she must loom over them like some sadistically happy, pony-tailed killing machine. I pity the bug who stumbles into Lucy's little screened-in bug house. (Right now there's a wooly bear caterpillar and some hapless pill bugs doing time on death row.)

Sometimes my heart goes out to the less revolting ones, and I'll bust them out when she's not looking. But if she catches me, she will sob like her dog died or something.

This girl needs a pet. *(Author's note: This piece was written well before I caved and invited a ridiculous menagerie of animals into our home.)*

But for now, this makeshift bug zoo will have to do.

Just this week, she bounded over and said, "Mommy, come see my museum!"

Scattered all over the garage floor was every plastic deli meat container I'd ever owned, and under each one was a different varmint—centipedes, slugs, ladybugs, roly-polies (whose disturbing real name, I've just learned, is woodlouse). She had curated quite a show, and she was rightfully proud.

I couldn't help but be puzzled over how this kid—whose heart soars at the sensation of worms in her hand—could be mine.

Truth be told, sometimes it's life's greatest joy (and relief) to see the ways my kids have turned out absolutely nothing like me.

Brave? Undaunted? Curious about what's under every rock? That's *so* not me—but I love that it's my daughter.

Because if Lucy isn't afraid to grab a slug by the tail, maybe she won't be afraid to grab life by the tail either.

Even if it does sometimes leave a pesky trail of slime.

Macchio Macchio Man
March 2013

Let's play a quick word association game.

You say, "karate." I say, what?

Ralph Macchio? Hong Kong Fooey? Concrete log splitting with your noggin?

I'll tell you what words *never once* sprang to mind: "Tuesdays and Thursdays, 5:15 p.m."

I'm as surprised as anyone to report that my nine-year-old indoor enthusiast has joined (am I using this word right?) a dojo.

He's even got the little white outfit to prove it—emblazoned with a gigantic cobra with an eagle's wings across the back.

I never saw this coming.

Will hasn't exactly been our resident All-Star, and that's okay. While he's dabbled in soccer and baseball, we've struggled mightily to land on something Will would dig doing just to have a more well-rounded life.

The Lego table is a wonderful place to visit. I just don't want my son to *live* there.

Will has rejected just about every possibility Western parents could dream up for their children's betterment—sailing lessons, guitar, hockey, basketball, Boy Scouts, lacrosse, art lessons, even the Junior Engineering program after school (which is based *entirely* on Legos). You can see what we're up against here.

If any one of those ideas pushed even the teeniest sliver of one pinky toenail out of Will's comfort zone, there was still no convincing him.

Before we could even get out the words—"Hey! This underwater penny-stacking class on Tuesdays looks interesting!"—he'd have flow charts prepared with every potentially applicable excuse.

I'd started to permanently unfurl the white flag when karate popped up on our radar screen.

Will's little buddy (who shares his lack of an "eye of the tiger") surprised us by signing up for a karate class. In a handful of lessons, he'd finally figured out his right from his left, how to jump rope, plus a few cool moves. His parents were thrilled. So was the kid.

This could be *it*, I thought. At karate, he'd have a friend to goof around with while working on some mad ninja skills at the same time. I may not know a sensei from a samurai sword, but I was sold.

Will, of course, was not.

When we suggested with great hopefulness that he try it out, his actual words to me were—and I quote—"This is the worst punishment you could ever dream up for me!"

This fun banter went on for quite a while. After he went to bed that night, I'll be honest: I cried. A lot.

Playing this never-ending tug-of-war with my child gets exhausting, but maybe even more so is the tug-of-war with myself. My internal warring factions kept going back and forth, and I had no idea who to root for.

One side of me wanted nothing more than for our kid to find something he loved *on his own*, to embrace it happily and with gusto. But the other side of me knows my kid well enough to see (because he's just like me) sometimes the only way forward is a forced march.

Without nudging him out of the nest once in a while, he might hunker down here forever—wasting a perfectly good set of wings he'd never learned to use.

So I made him try karate two days later. And I'm proud to say, he judo-chopped, he played dodge ball, he laughed at the sensei's jokes. Like Mikey and that age-old bowl of cereal, he liked it. He actually liked it.

I wrote out a check before the kid could change his mind.

I had to. This could be Will's only chance to learn how to catch flies with chopsticks.

And you just don't turn down an opportunity like that.

A Chip is to Queso as a Tent is to _____ (and No, the Answer Isn't "Being Murdered in the Woods")

July 2015

Don't be confused. The minute I get one of those Patagonia catalogs with someone striking a yoga pose atop Machu Picchu, I don't think twice. I don't flip through the pages longingly. I don't even hesitate.

I toss it straight in the trash without a backward glance at their wide array of sports bras.

My soul does *not* yearn for adventure. Or exertion. Or going more than twenty-four hours without God's gift of showering.

But I just spent the weekend in a tent with my family. And you know what? I could very well do it again.

Oddly enough, all that fresh air and togetherness was—I can't believe I'm saying this—*good for us.*

The only screen was the fire, which everyone stared at like it was Facebook. The only chores were the half-assed kind of dishwashing that happens with cold water and a laissez-faire camping attitude. The only to-do items involved very little adult participation, like capturing every moth that dared draw near our lantern or creating a mud puddle island retreat for a new lizard friend.

It wasn't Norman Rockwell idyllic. Nothing ever is, *really.*

There was a lot of swearing and snapping as my husband and I fumbled to recall how to pitch this god-forsaken tent. In the dark.

There was feverish swatting at whatever Deep Woods Off! wouldn't ward off.

There was zero sleep when our nightmare-plagued girl shoehorned her way onto our narrow, sinking air mattress. (We don't sleep on the ground, people. What are we, savages?)

There was a huge bug bite on my husband's arm that got all swollen and angry, much like the spider with bloody fangs that caused it while attempting to kill us in our sleep.

Then there was the time I grabbed at a teetering lantern and burned my fingertips to a bacony crisp. (This was essentially my first act of camping—eradicating my fingerprints.)

But I am choosing to look at it this way: just as the nacho chip is the ho-hum vehicle for enjoying the awesomeness of queso, the tent shall be our cheap vehicle for finding awesomeness out in the world together.

This weekend, that tent was our cleanliness-challenged jumping off point for seeing the Berkshires (where I'd never been), checking out a fancy-pants art museum (in a greasy ponytail not quite in keeping with the Lilly Pulitzer vibe), and then consuming a platter of random meaty deliciousness at our very first Colombian restaurant.

Not half bad for life from a tent.

I have to say, we just do better out there.

In our house, the husband and I are on task. We have things to do. We get distracted and crabby and want to be left alone to our projects, our solitude, or our three-hundredth viewing of *A Few Good Men* on TBS. We growl and shoo the kids off to a screen of their own.

But *out there*, even if we're in a tent, we're together on purpose. We have plans. We are lighter in our spirit. We may be cheap (hence the tent), but we're up for stuff.

And I cannot stress to you what a miracle this is . . . out there, from that tent, our children played together a) outside, and b) without arguing.

These baby vampires—who shriek at the very suggestion that they should *go outside and play*—spent hours collecting a plastic container full of weird swamp monster newts then throwing a "party" for them in a shady spot by the lake.

Anybody want second helpings of that? *Yes, please.*

If it takes a tent for us all to get outside of the house and outside of ourselves, consider me draped in nylon and bug spray and halfway out the door.

Together—our fists full of tent stakes, our hair slick with sheen, our hearts swelling with adventure—we will go out and see the world.

Mosquitos, Lyme disease, and body odor be damned.

PART V

WELCOME TO ESTROGEN COUNTRY

Womanhood is a weird place to be.

I realized just *how weird* when I was trying to explain to my growing-up girl about (enter full-body shudder) menstruation.

Let's just say, she was *stunned* to learn that this crap goes on.

It was kind of awful to talk about (and by "talk," I mean, the act of grasping for words—and air—while shoving American Girl's *The Care and Keeping of You* at her).

For her sake, I wished she wouldn't have to learn her way around a plastic applicator or worry about red dots creeping onto white leggings. Short-sighted though it may be, we moms want nothing but good tidings for our girls, and decades of visits from a bloated, leaky, achy "monthly friend" does *not* neatly fit that category.

I know, I know. There's a bigger, more glorious purpose to it all. And yeah, yeah, we are fearfully and wonderfully made and all that. I get it. I *do*. God's whole master plan works amazingly well most of the time. But still . . . *yuck*.

Girls just have their own special brand of weird stuff to deal with.

And as girls, we love to talk our girl stuff to death. Sometimes I even want to write lots of words about girl stuff (like I've done in this section). And yes, every now and then, I even get cranky about girl stuff.

But if you're a man reading this, I suggest you steer clear of the obvious question. Let's just go ahead and assume the answer is yes.

It *is* that time of the month.

The Day the Mom Jeans Died
May 2012

Congratulate me. I am the proud owner of my first pair of skinny jeans.

Through a process of attrition and creeping waistline growth, I'd gotten myself down to one pair of jeans—one desperately sad pair of dowdy mom-cut jeans, sagging in the rear and giving off a distinct vibe of defeat.

No one who beheld my baggy behind could miss the white flag these jeans were waving.

"Here sits a woman of once relative attractiveness," my jeans would say. "She's all done with that now. Come! Follow us to Chico's!"

I had looked at my sad backside in the mirror one too many times, so on Mother's Day afternoon, I resolved to do something about it.

I headed to the Gap, squeezed myself into a dark rinse pair of skinny jeans, and a la Olivia Newton-John at the end of *Grease*—I was reborn.

Okay, maybe it wasn't as transformative as a Lycra catsuit. Still, I considered it a victorious baby step off the destructive path leading to mix-and-match poly-blend separates.

Just that morning, eight-year-old Will served me breakfast in bed. With my cheese Danish, I was presented with a mock newspaper he'd made at school, emblazoned with the headline "World's Best Mom!"

The sidebar offered a handy checklist that read, "My Mother is . . . (check all that apply)."

Now, I have to ask: what defect in my nature caused me to skim right past all the perfectly lovely qualities my son checked off about me to get to the ones he *didn't*?

I mean, the last I heard, there wasn't a thing wrong with "brilliant," "funny," or even "cuddly."

But with my mental highlighter pen, I honed in like a tractor beam on the unchecked "brave." On "cute." On "energetic." (The kid had me there.) And hey, what gives? I didn't rank a "wise"?

At least he had the good sense to check "pretty." Skipping that one can only lead to misery—an apt lesson for any man to learn from an early age.

This checklist cranked the volume on the voice in my head that'd been whispering, "You're being watched. Are you someone worth watching?"

For too long, my kids have been a convenient scapegoat for my slovenliness. Once upon a time, there were years I cared a little too intensely about how I looked—from the days of poring over fashion magazines in despair to the grown-up angst of getting a man down the aisle. Then came a welcomed period of sloth when a paunchy midriff could be blamed on a baby. And eventually, so could spit-up-encrusted sweaters and Sharpie-stained chinos until *nothing* became my fault.

I was a *mom*. (Sigh.) Nothing more could possibly be expected of me.

But now my kids are eight and six, and I'm realizing that the "me" I present to the world—and the attitude toward life that this "me" represents—has the potential to affect my children. To embarrass them. To rub off on them. To inspire them—or not.

I'm the first to say life's not all about appearances. Lord knows I hate the idea of my daughter being consumed by what *Cosmo Girl* tells her she should be. But for me, it's about owning up to the fact that I am a role model for my kids—probably the most important one.

And while I'll never check off every item on the World's Best Mom list, I still want to show my kids a person worth emulating—preferably a "wise" woman who "bravely" and "energetically" shows up for life.

And with a few sit-ups now and then, possibly even a mom who's "cute" doing it.

Living Out Loud
(I Mean, Really, Really Loud)

April 2009

Chatty Cathy. If there was ever a national symbol of jaw jacking, she's it. But even at her most verbose, Chatty Cathy knew when to quit. Eighteen happy little phrases, and she was *done*.

Three-year-old Lucy is a charming Kewpie doll of a girl—but she's one with no word limit, no string to pull, and definitely no pause button. I swear, these days the child *never stops talking*.

We always knew there was a lot going on inside that head. Even from the high chair, the kid would create entire scenes of dialogue between two Mini-Wheats.

But what was once quietly contained is now spilling over into the world. And man, is it loud.

She is finding her voice, which means that if my son has something to tell me about his day at preschool (a coveted and rare conversation indeed), she will have something to tell me *louder*. Cutting her brother off mid-sentence, she'll inch closer to my face and insist, "Mommy, let's talk about *my* school!"

Never mind the fact that she doesn't *go* to school. Details . . .

Lucy wants to be heard, and woe to you if she's not. Being ignored has become a fate worse than death (or at least worse than a hangnail), which is unfortunate since Will has inherited an uncanny set of ignoring skills from his father.

It's nearly a daily occurrence to hear Will protest in great exasperation, "But I don't want to *talk*, Lucy!" (He is, after all, a male person limited to a finite number of words a day.)

Then comes the wailing, her head thrown back, mouth open in a stricken moan.

"He said he doesn't want to play with *meee!*"

In mournful moments like these, Lucy hikes up not just the volume, but the octave. We lovingly refer to this as "Beaker Mode" as she morphs into the Muppets' googly-eyed lab assistant—wailing an unintelligible and high-pitched "Me, me, me, meee!" as if her lab coat's on fire.

But the newest manifestation of her verbosity is Lucy as comedienne. I guess she's figuring out that around these parts, the best way to be heard is to lead with a joke.

So now she's busy making up terrible knock-knock jokes, rewriting song lyrics into musical Mad Libs, and twisting her face into maniacal grins when she wants to weasel back into my good graces.

She's especially adept at mimicry, best known for copying the inflections of Sylvester from *Loony Toons* to lispy perfection. You can imagine our pride when she asked her Sunday School teacher in a Sylvester-ish snarl, "What are ya looking for, a chapped lip?" (The cat actually says "fat" lip, but I don't know . . . maybe chapped lips are worse.)

Hers is a madcap little mind, and it's entertaining to gain a better view inside. At the same time, all this gum flapping can jangle the nerves, never having a moment of quiet to reflect on solutions to world hunger or ring around the collar.

I'll say this for the girl: at least she's speaking a language I understand. Will is a boy. And as such, he will remain an eternal mystery to me. I have literally no idea what goes on his male mind.

But dramatic? Whiny? Desperate to be heard, to score the laugh, to connect, to be understood?

That, I get.

That, I *am*.

What Lies Beneath: What Mammograms and Motherhood Reveal

March 2012

Christy doesn't *seem* like the name of a sadist.

Yet there she was, squishing my already flat and unmentionable lady parts in a vice and taking pictures. It reminded me of a scene in *Casino*—except, thank God, Joe Pesci wasn't there.

Welcome to my first mammogram.

I honestly didn't think what Christy did to me (in her pert ponytail and purple scrubs) was humanly possible—that a) she could find something capable of mashing, and b) that she could manage to spread out that something so far and wide that I'd actually want to take a picture as proof.

Just one of the wonders of technology, I suppose—and one of the many mortifications of getting old.

Like buying your first box of Clairol Nice 'n' Easy or watching *Masterpiece Theatre*, it's all part of the growing-up process—a process that kicks into humiliating high gear the moment you start making babies.

Speaking of which, this particular mammography joint was right next door to the doctor's office where I'd stood in soggy-bottomed maternity pants after my water broke eight years earlier.

Not much is grosser—or more utterly life-changing—than that.

Pregnancy and childbirth can't help but transform us in deep and meaningful ways. We blossom into completeness. We feel poised to fulfill our destinies. We get weirdly nonchalant about God and every-body being all up in our private parts.

This is coming from a modest mouse who used to experience heart palpitations at the phrase *pap smear* and had stopped wearing bikinis by age nine.

But after birthing two children—a process in which every be-scrubbed lackey in the Tri-State Area seemed to take a gander at my nether-regions—I became a hardened professional. I'd fling my legs into those stirrups week after week like a boss, chatting away about the weather with the top of my doctor's head.

It's degrading stuff, but you get over it.

That's motherhood for ya.

———————

From the putting-it-all-out-there moment when a baby comes screeching out of you, parenting just keeps right on stripping you bare in front of everybody.

Once and for all, parenting ends the charade.

It exposes who you really are.

And might I suggest that those real selves likely include (but are not limited to) the following:

You're a yeller; you're neurotic, you're a germophobe; you're a social climber; you're selfish; you've got a short fuse; you have no interest in playing on the floor; you're peevish; you're scared of *everything* (e.g., online predators, SIDS, raw cake batter, dust mites, drunk babysitters, uncut grapes, flights of stairs, conversion vans . . . all of it).

And, oh yeah, you have absolutely no idea what you're doing.

All the things you thought you weren't because you hid them so well? Trust me, *you are.*

And since you'd somehow managed not to broadcast all your issues to the world before motherhood, your kids are just thoughtful enough to drag them all into the light *for you*—usually in public, and almost always in the grocery store check-out lane.

It's not pretty, but it's probably what has to happen for us to fully acquire "grown-up" status.

Besides, if my mammogram didn't light up those few weird little things, I would never know they were there and might need fixing.

And if parenting didn't shine a daily light on all my deepest flaws, I'd never be forced to face them and start rooting them out so that a kinder, gentler, better version of myself could emerge.

Granted, I haven't seen that kinder, gentler me yet, but she's got to be around here somewhere. . . .

A Head-Banging Case
of the "Hey, Mom"s

June 2011

"Hey, Mom."

Those two words sound innocent enough. Not inherently evil. Not particularly bothersome. Maybe even kind of sweet.

But if you multiply those two little words by . . . I don't know . . . a *jillion* times a day, "Hey, Mom" (now seven-year-old Will's go-to conversation starter) is a phrase capable of leading a mother down a very dark path.

In 99.9 percent of cases, "Hey, Mom" results in adverse Pavlovian reactions, e.g., full-body twitching, eye-rolling, room-bolting, and (after prolonged use) stark raving madness.

In layman's terms, the "Hey, Mom"s are making me insane.

Really and truly, the phrase "Hey, Mom" might not be so bad if there were some exclamation marks thrown in. At least then my kid might come off like a jolly Kool-Aid Man who just can't help busting through walls to tell me something fantastic.

Or maybe I could even handle it if "Hey, Mom" didn't always come with that *excruciating* pause.

But there's always this weird time lapse after every "Hey, Mom," as though he's waiting for me to look up, make meaningful eye contact, and respond with giddy anticipation: "Yes, dear child, I am in rapt attention about the special features on your Nerf gun. Do tell me more!"

There's only so many times you can hear "Hey, Mom" before you figure out this arresting little phrase merely gives the *appearance* of urgency. There's never blood. No one is ever on fire (which, I suppose, is a good thing).

"Hey, Mom" is just the handiest interruption of whatever monumental thing I was doing, saying, or shopping online for so my child can get back to sharing whatever vital, unfiltered thought just passed through the transoms of his mind.

As a general rule, the "Hey, Mom"s are almost always a) nonsensical, b) a million miles off any topic I was talking about or would *ever* talk about, or c) Lego-related.

———

To paint a clearer picture for you, let me share a few "Hey, Mom" examples from just this past week. (I did *not* make these up.)

"Hey, Mom . . ."(long pause) "Did you know that Master Shifu (the one with the mustache in *Kung Fu Panda*) can stand on one foot for two whole minutes?"

"Hey, Mom . . . I made this Lego speeder so it can go underwater."

"Hey, Mom . . . Do you know what my favorite restaurant is? Longhorn. They have the best steak and H1N1 Sauce." (That's what he once called A1 Sauce during the height of flu season. I thought it was hysterical, so we will never call it anything else.)

"Hey, Mom . . . I know what 'nine' is in Spanish? *Nueve.*" (Bonus points for actually sharing something he learned in school.)

"Hey, Mom . . . I'm gonna tell you something I never told anyone—I really want a barracuda stuffed animal."

"Hey, Mom . . . I know you're not gonna like this, but is it okay if I get started on my Christmas list?" (It's *June.*)

But here's the one that makes me want to stab my eyes out with the nearest mechanical pencil—mainly because it's the single most overused "Hey, Mom" of all time and is almost always accompanied by irksome amounts of lurking. Every mother in the civilized world knows this one intimately and dreads its appearance.

"Hey Mom . . . Whatcha doing?"

Sigh. This is the "Hey, Mom" of summer.

———

On one hand, there are obviously some social skills we need to work on here. The boy has to learn that it's rude to blurt out that he changed his mind and really wants the Lego Cad Bane Speeder more than the Mandalorian Battle Pack—right smack in the middle of my earth-shattering conversation with my husband about whether that second *Hangover* movie should have ever happened.

On the other hand, it's rude of me to automatically discount everything coming out of my child's mouth just because so many of his thoughts seem to have launched from Planet Nine.

He has a voice. His thoughts have value. And even if my son and I look at the world through very different lenses, he has important things to share with me.

Things like "Hey, Mom. You look pretty today."

Obviously nonsensical and untrue, but hey, let the kid talk.

From Glass Slippers to Go-Go Boots—How to Keep the Fairy Tale from Fracturing

May 2008

At our house, everything's gone royal.

From Her Majesty's plastic throne (a.k.a. her high chair), two-year-old Lucy rules over an enchanted land where shriveled pieces of morning sausage become "princesses" and a row of used party hats becomes a castle. It's not uncommon to catch her fork and spoon waltzing at a royal ball.

In this land, she calls every frock in her closet a "Cinderella," and a decree has gone forth that these are to be Lucy's standard uniform. On days when I fail to adorn her in the "proper raiment," I can usually find her with a tutu cinched up over her footie pajamas.

It is cuteness with a capital "C" (or "K" for those who like those "klever" spellings).

But this Princess Syndrome can also produce its share of cringe-worthy moments—like when Lucy beams at herself in the mirror and says, "I'm a princess. I *boo-ful*."

I'm all for having a healthy sense of self—but I'd like to steer clear of the narcissistic kind that parades around in T-shirts that say "Diva!" or "Spoiled Rotten!" (Talk about a self-fulfilling prophecy . . .)

In addition to the perils of an over-inflated sense of royalty, we mothers of princess wannabes must do battle against the dreaded "damsel in distress" notion. As there may or may not be a rich, handsome prince coming to Lucy's rescue one day, she'd best learn to do more in her ivory tower free time than grow really long Crystal Gayle locks.

But my biggest worry in Princess Land is wondering where this golden road will lead. Sure, it starts out all nice and flat-chested with Snow White, but then you move on to a boy-crazy mermaid busting out of her shell bra. Next thing you know, Ariel's graduated to Malibu Barbie all dolled up and straight out of a plastic prostitution ring.

They actually make Barbies now with *tattoos*. Have you seen these? That prude Skipper has long been thrown overboard for a whole new posse of Barbies sporting go-go boots, diamond navel rings, and sparkly cell phones (probably for calling their pimps and not that kill-joy, Ken).

So if it's good enough for the new tatted-up Barbie, it's good enough for your kindergartner. Kiddie racks today are full of clothes that are clingy, low-rise, and suggestive enough to wear with pint-sized thong underwear. It's why I'm scared to death of trying to raise a girl in this world.

Our little princesses are being forced to grow up at break-neck speed. (Just ask Miley Cyrus.) Worse, they're growing into versions of young adulthood I don't even recognize—one replete with stripper poles, foul mouths, and boob jobs as graduation gifts.

So as I shake my old-fogey fist at MTV and mutter phrases like *hell in a hand basket,* I wonder to myself: How in the world do you do it? How do you raise a kind, smart, self-respecting young woman in a world of girls gone wild?

I assure you there's no shortage of strategies I'll try (not the least of which is big-time prayer). But one thing I'll do is stick my finger in this culture dam as hard as I can, while trying to download my little girl's big imagination with visions of what cool chicks *really* look like.

I'll start with a healthy dose of Laura Ingalls Wilder and Louisa May Alcott, a smattering of those old yellow-bound Nancy Drews, followed by a whole lot of Julie Andrews, Carol Burnett, and re-runs of *I Love Lucy.* When the time is right, she will know Tina and Amy, too.

After years of undaunted motherly brainwashing, the time will come for Lucy to leave Cinderella's castle. And when she does, my best hope is that my little princess will ignore the siren song of the Bratz Rock Angelz and the skanky pop divas and make her own merry way all the way to Sunnybrook Farm. Or 30 Rock. Whichever comes first.

Lordy, Lordy, Look Who's in Pajama Jeans

July 2011

It's my fortieth birthday, and I'll cry if I want to. (You would cry too if it happened to you.)

Maybe it already did and you've already had that cry. Maybe you know the feeling of getting dragged into this weird realm where we now feel a kinship with our sisters in half-glasses and elastic waistbands, where we actually entertain the thought of getting us a pair of those infomercial "pajama jeans," where folks our age start looking to Jamie Lee Curtis for tips on digestive health.

If this is you, come join me at the grown-up table. I just earned a permanent spot.

I can't promise you any wild parties here; we're way past that. Shoot, nobody at the grown-up table much bothers with birthdays anymore. That thrill died at twenty-one. (As did our days of shopping at places with names like Forever 21 . . . a store that didn't even exist when I was twenty-one. Sigh.)

Back when we were kids, there was no greater delight invented by man than a birthday. We'd no sooner get past one before we were counting down to the next. For children, birthdays are the ultimate sugar-spun celebration of self—a day where nothing else matters but *me*. Oh yeah, and presents. For *me*.

But most of us reach a certain point (maybe it was the discovery of a chin hair or underarms that jiggle when you clap) when we start seeing some downsides to this whole birthday thing. And after forty of them celebrated on planet Earth, we can't help but grow a little mellower, a little wiser, and a little less inclined to smash piñatas.

I don't know about you, but all I really want at this point is a babysitter.

And so (unlike my preteen self, circa 1982), it didn't take a slumber party with a trampoline to make my forty-year-old birthday wishes come true. All it took was dinner for two at a grown-up restaurant, a small box in my husband's hand (always a good sign it's not a blender), and a chocolate confection that someone else baked waiting for us back home.

There may not have been a bouncy castle in the yard, but considering my advanced age and my perilously low calcium intake, that's a good thing.

Whatever. I'm old. It's official. I'm okay with it.

So stop by the grown-up table next time you're in the neighborhood. We can't promise laser tag, but we'll have chocolate and cloth napkins and hopefully a growing supply of emotional maturity tucked away in our wrinkly creases.

I'll be easy to spot. I'll be the one in the faux-denim stretch pants.

PART VI

HOLIDAYS, VACATIONS, AND OTHER NATURAL DISASTERS

I've written a lot about holidays and vacations—maybe more than any other topic—because I just can't *not*. These life events are so big and overstuffed—with meaning, pressure, drama, and complex (that's my nice word) characters who may or may not reside in our family tree.

Holidays and family vacays are just *a lot*.

Against any measure of good sense and decent gas mileage, these brouhahas call on us to cram the Family Truckster to the brink of disaster with children, pets, coolers, gifts, Chex Mix, tents, baby gear, boogie boards, bikes, DVD players, pillows, craft supplies, Capri Suns, pent-up anxieties, a good bit of emotional baggage, way too much actual baggage, and everything else gets strapped to the top with bungee cords. (For your sake, I hope this excludes dearly departed loved ones.)

We also like to strap onto these big life events some staggeringly high expectations. We look forward to our summers and family travels and holidays for what seems like millennia. We make bigger than normal plans for them. We spend tons of money on them. We buy new clothes and dress up for them—sometimes even subjecting ourselves to the horrors of swimsuit shopping in preparation for them.

And every once in a beautiful while, that thing you planned for like a doomsday prepper delivers in a big way; the skies open and a host of angels sing for glory. That's the stuff we live for. This is the shy, rare, magical unicorn of family life.

But sometimes the thing that sounded so lovely on paper ends up sucking the life out of you with all its schlepping and whining and interpersonal chafing, and all you want to do is go home with a carton of spiked egg nog and sleep it off. So we write that one off and hope for better luck next year. This is the irritating, energy-sucking tsetse fly of family life.

Lastly (and maybe best of all), sometimes the big thing is a total train wreck. Sometimes that summer "getaway" in the spider-infested cabin or that disastrous Thanksgiving when the dog ate the turkey falls so spectacularly short that it becomes the stuff of epic storytelling for generations. This is the crazy drunken phoenix rising from the ashes of family life. It was so legendarily bad that you will laugh about it until your dying day. At the time, there was nothing worse. But in the long run, there's nothing better.

Just try not to let your dying day happen on vacation. It'll bum everybody out. Plus, there's no more room in, under, or on top of this car for any more dead relatives.

Sixty-Eight Days of Summer, and One in Every Crowd

June 2015

Stretching before us are sixty-eight days of summer vacation. *Sixty-eight*.

That is many, many days, my friends.

And let me warn you right now, there will be *one*. In every family, on every road trip, on every outing of perfectly planned frivolity:

There will be one who sulks.

There will be one who never stops talking.

There will be one who wants to do *everything*.

There will be one who wants to do *nothing*.

There will be one who won't quit begging for snacks.

There will be one who asks a zillion questions about what we're doing next, what we'll do there, when we're going *home*.

There will be one who doesn't like hot dogs.

There will be one who doesn't want his face getting wet.

There will be one who straggles behind.

There will be one who is bored.

There will be one whose bladder is always bursting.

There will be one who hates the movie that everyone else loves.

There will be one who gets carsick.

There will be one who needlessly pokes at his siblings in the backseat.

There will be one who spills her Slurpee into the seat cushions.

There will be one who refuses to sleep in a tent, use a porta-potty, wear the swimmies . . . fill in the blank.

There will be one who wants to stay in the pool when everyone else wants to go to the ocean.

There will be one who wants to go to the ocean when everyone else wants to stay in the pool.

There will be one who is eternally hangry.

There will be one who leaves behind the single most important thing ever in the history of mankind (be it a favorite stuffed animal, flip-flops, or the can't-live-without gadget of the moment).

There will be one who is cold.

There will be one who is hot.

There will always be *one* in every crowd.

As we throw ourselves headlong into summer, we would all be wise to remember this simple truth: there will always be *one*.

It's as inevitable as the summer buzz of mosquitos. Yes, mosquitos are annoying as fire, but when they come, somehow we are not undone by this news. We mildly swat at them. We light citronella candles that don't work. We stock up on DEET and Skin-So-Soft and try to ward them off as best we can.

But we know this to be true: the mosquitos will always be among us. We don't get all huffy about it. We just try to endure them and make the best of our shared airspace anyway.

Our kids are not *mosquitos*. They are dear sweet precious gifts from heaven above (ahem), but at any given moment, one of them will be buzzing with unhappiness when everyone else is just peachy.

I say: Whatevs.

Press on.

Give that kid a granola bar and your best fake smile and crank up the radio.

We are together.

We are making some happy freaking memories.

We will enjoy the view anyway . . . dive in the water anyway . . . hike to the top anyway . . . check out that cute shop anyway. Because everybody else wants to and we are *pressing the heck on.*

———————

I'm preaching to myself more than I'm preaching to you, because I know myself and my sky-high expectations. I am never quite prepared for *the one* who is intent on ruining the picture-perfect slide show in my head by being hungry, cranky, loud, whiney, injured, bored, *whatever*.

But it's just not possible for everyone to be *psyched* all the time, to like all the same things, to love everything I suggest, to perform perfectly on cue. This summer, I will resolve not to take it personally, not to get all naggy and ranty and pouty when *the one* shows up.

Sometimes—I'm man enough to admit it—*I* am *the one*.

Yet we press on, knowing that eventually *the one* will get with the program. Get a protein fix. Catch up. Get caught smiling. Make fun memories anyhow. It'll be worth it.

And after we have soldiered our way through all sixty-eight days of family fun, I will be rewarded with a camera full of sunny memories—and yes, a hard-earned backpack full of school supplies.

So let's go out and make some memories already—even if *the one* shows up.

Even if it kills us.

Yuletide Greetings from Our Cozy Connecticut Estate to Yours

December 2012

Our family Christmas card this year is in dire need of a disclaimer.

In fine print under the warm seasonal greetings, it ought to read: "Objects in these phony-baloney photographs are crankier, sloppier, poorer, and more plagued by nagging existential angst than they appear."

I don't mean to brag, but our Christmas card photos turned out really good this year . . . maybe a little *too* good.

I'm afraid we're going to give our friends the wrong impression—first, that we live at Downton Abbey (the pictures were taken at an honest-to-God *mansion*); and secondly, that we're living some picture-perfect, Facebook-ready life—one where we are always sporting matching clothes, effortless smiles, and boundless *joie de vivre*.

Don't believe everything you see.

A friend who's starting a photography venture took our pictures this year. When she asked to use us as guinea pigs for her portfolio, I happily gave my tripod the year off.

She just might have outdone herself.

Plunking us down in an idyllic Connecticut setting with most of our hairs in place, we were transformed from a rag-tag band of Clampetts into the Family Hilfiger, frolicking in roll-neck sweaters at our cozy Hamptons estate.

Allow me to set the scene. (Spoiler alert: It's a-dorable!).

There are my darling children, holding hands as they run across the mansion lawn. Now watch them blow soap flakes into the air in a whimsical poof of holiday "snow." See the family matriarch (that's me) wearing something woolen and J.Crew—consignment J.Crew on clearance, but J.Crew nonetheless. See how the patriarch's plaid ties us all together with perfect shades of Christmas crimson. It's enough to make the whole world sing.

Please hear me when I say—this is not reality. This is the work of a professional.

I've thought about sending out a follow-up card in the style of those "Stars Without Makeup!" tabloid covers—just to keep it real. I'm envisioning a photo collage showcasing what we *actually* look like day-to-day, complete with those awful black arrows to provide a handy field guide of our flaws.

One arrow would point out my non-pregnant "baby bump" from beneath an unflattering hoodie. Another could highlight Lucy's flaming circle of lip chap speckled with ketchup and leftover lunch. A third arrow could point to Will's ribs poking through his T-shirt as he pouts over another untouched dinner plate. We'd need at least one more arrow to showcase the wisps of steam shooting from Dad's ears in the next chair.

A whole quiver full of arrows would be needed to expose this house's secret squalor—floors so littered with Legos or laundry you have to pole vault your way across, dog hair taking on the form of a shag rug in certain sectors I ignore, random towers of paper that may never, ever see a folder or filing cabinet.

But here's the kicker. Those arrows can't even begin to show the hot mess we are *inside*. Let's just say, it's not all merry and bright. That's the ugly truth for our family—and for anyone who's ever sent a happy family Christmas card photo out into the world.

We all love our families. And we'd all love for family life to be as delightful as it seems in front of this sand dune/glowing tree/stately mansion.

But we all know that as soon as that shutter closes, someone will cry, fight, or trip headlong over a rogue piece of driftwood. We'll be tired. We'll yell. We may end up in the ER. And we'll be frustrated that our family seems much more akin to the Island of Misfit Toys than those unrecognizable, pretty people in the picture.

But who on my Christmas card list really wants to see how our family sausage is made? Nobody, that's who. Behind the scenes, it gets ugly, chaotic, and our outfits don't even match.

But the end result of sausage-making is *sausage*, and sausage is good. So let's just stick with *that*.

Our family is one heck of a mess to make, but it's made with love and a heaping helping of God's grace.

And maybe this Christmas and every Christmas, that's all you need to know.

My Own Private *SS Minnow*
July 2010

You picked a fine time to leave me, Ma Bell.

Here it is, the dead calm of summer. Nobody's around except my two kids, shadowing me with expectant looks and requests for snacks. And of all my lonely and desperate hours, *this* is the time our phone line decided to go on the fritz.

Talking on the phone in its current state sounds like I'm inside the microwave with Orville Redenbacher, so there's no way to call anybody. Worse, whatever devilry's making all that crackling also means I can't get on the Internet, can't email, and can't escape my current reality to electronically peek at what's happening in yours.

The phrase *trapped on a desert island* has become part of my daily ranting and raving. Life here is starting to look a whole lot like *Gilligan's Island*.

By default (as the only sane person present), I'm the Professor. I'm the castaway-in-charge, the one everyone looks to for new and exciting escape plans. (Those plans are typified by feverish planning, the occasional monkey, and spectacular failure.)

I've even started to wear the Professor's haunted expression—the one that silently pleads to all passers-by: "Help me. I'm surrounded by crazy people and head hunters."

Now it sure is sweet of you to think such a thing, but no, I couldn't possibly be *Ginger*.

Farmer's tan, tree stump thighs, frumpy mom tankini—none of that adds up to a Ginger. (I am also very poorly coiffed.) Sadly, there's no Ginger here—nor any semblance of gold lamé. Let's just skip her.

The real trick in this desert island scenario is deciding which parts my *kids* are playing.

Sometimes they're all Thurston and Lovey—a pampered pair that was quite sure their three-hour tour was going to be way more fun than this. They need a full-time travel agent to entertain their every summer whim.

Sometimes they're every bit the Skipper and Gilligan—bumbling buddies trapped in a state of love-hate. Theirs is a constant loop of growling, groaning, and head-clunking, followed by complaints lodged with the Professor over the irritating things Gilligan has done or said now.

But lots of days, Lucy doubles as our resident Mary Ann, all sunny contentment and bouncing curls, wearied by all the grumpiness on this stupid island.

Then there's my husband, who plays one of those random guest-stars who just magically shows up on the island—a Harlem Globetrotter of sorts. He flits in and out, making nice, friendly appearances to keep things interesting. Then—poof!—he gets to return to civilization while here we sit, stuck with a hole in our boat, no new ideas, and no place to go.

Being a Globetrotter is good.

Don't get me wrong. Desert island living has its perks.

The pace is easy. You don't have to be anywhere on time. You can wear the same pants every day and nobody knows the difference.

And if you're really living right, sometimes there's even time to kick back with a coconut drink—as long as you can tune out the ruckus behind you of Gilligan and the Skipper squabbling their way out of that wretched hammock one more time.

Visits from the Ghosts of Halloween Past, Present, and Future

October 2010

Almost every Halloween of my childhood, I wore the snoozer of all costumes: I was a ghost in a sheet.

On my face was a rickety Casper mask held together with yellowing Scotch tape. The rest of me was covered in a white sheet on which my mom had traced a picture of that perky poltergeist in Magic Marker. Every October thirty-first of my memory, Mom threw this sheet over my head and called it a day.

I'm pretty sure if there had been a *Star Search* scorecard for my Halloween performance, Ed McMahon would have bellowed in great disappointment: "Zero and a quarter stars!"

In this age of great craftiness, I've often looked back and snarked about what a dud that costume was and how unimaginative my mother was for making me wear it. But after going 'round and 'round with my four-year-old about what she's going to be this Halloween, I've started to cut my mom some slack.

First of all, and most importantly, it was the seventies. Nobody gave a crap.

Second of all, what if those Casper re-runs weren't entirely Mom's doing? What if she'd *tried* to come up with something a little snappier, but it was *me* who shut her down? Now that I've got kids of my own, I'm starting to see how this works.

For weeks, I've been feeding Lucy a mile-long list of genius costume ideas, and she's poo-poo'd every last one. I've been standing at the ready to engineer the perfect Princess Leia buns, to scour Goodwill for the perfect shreddable Frankenstein blazer, to transform any cardboard edifice into a Lego block, unicorn, or Crayola crayon.

But all she wants to be is what she was last year: a fairy ballerina.

Girl, *please*. That is *so* last season.

I guess I ought to be relieved she doesn't want a bloody butcher knife duct-taped to her head. It's just that I get these ideas stuck in my brain of what my kids should do and think (e.g., You should learn guitar so you can lead campfire sing-alongs! You should love wearing that monogrammed jumper! You should hate all movies with talking Chihuahuas!)

It's weird, but my kids don't dig my ideas nearly as much as I do. Or *at all*.

Could it be possible—and I'm just spit-balling here—that my children aren't formless blobs to be molded into *my* image? I get so used to bossing them around that I forget God made them individuals with their own quirks, dreams, and ideas—ideas that don't always walk in contented lockstep with mine.

I'll give you an example from *somebody else's* family, which goes to show I'm not the only one who does this. I have a friend whose kindergarten daughter looks like a blonde angel floating on a cloud. And for this angelic daughter, Mother bought Daughter a darling little ladybug costume—a perfectly sweet vision of how Mother sees Daughter. Of course, Daughter revolted and sent Mother back to the store with her receipt. This angel wanted to be (what else?) *a devil*. A glittery little she-devil, complete with bedazzled horns and pitchfork.

Ladybug versus she-devil. I would like to refrain from using the expression *enough said*. But seriously, *enough said*.

———

In our parental mind's eye, we sketch out all these intricate designs and plans of what we want our children to be. Then they blow up our dreamy imaginings and come up with their own versions of them-selves—ones that are sometimes radically, always uniquely, but entirely their own.

This battle of wills began when those babies came bursting out of their swaddled-up hospital blankets, tiny fists of fury blazing. And it'll keep on going until I'm wagging a calcium-depleted finger at them, "advising" them on how to raise their own children.

I'll always have my own ideas (which will be *amazing*, of course). Some they'll ignore, some will stick. Oddly enough, they'll have their own ideas, too. Some will be dumb. And some will be the best ever.

But when my children show up at the pearly gates in whatever crazy patchwork get-ups they've put together in this life, my greatest prayer is that they'll have left lives full of love behind them, they'll have hearts full of faith inside them, and they'll have one heck of a snazzy crown of jewels waiting for them.

And yes, I pray they hear those precious words we all long to hear: "Three and three-quarter stars!"

It may not be perfection, but Ed McMahon, Saint Peter, and I will surely be very proud.

It's Summer. A Motherly MacGyver Must Rise Up.

July 2015[1]

Every spring, as we moms drag ourselves toward the school-year finish line, we greet each other with the same bleary-eyed refrain: "How long till summer?"

We smirk, give a half-hearted sigh, and shuffle away—the staggering, groaning *Walking Dead*–like shells of the A+ moms we once were, having long lost the will to sign reading logs or bring in allergen-free class snacks. From the tattered remains of our three-quarter-length sleeves, we strain our zombie arms toward the light . . . toward the carefree, sun-kissed days of summer.

Oh, but my dear, sweet, deluded ones, can't you see that's just the fog of war talking? We have forgotten what summer can be like.

Worse, we have forgotten that *children* will be there.

———

When my kids were in their early elementary years, I'd look ahead to summer—not with the wistful longing of the battle-weary, but with a paper bag affixed to my lips.

I remember having startling conversations with mothers of older kids who'd say nutty stuff like, "Man, I cannot *wait* for summer!"

These people faced the prospect of summer with *genuine good cheer*. I was dumbfounded. I remember contorting my face into a look of

———

1 This one blends several columns I've written about summer from June 2012, July 2008, and July 2013.

"Yeah, me too!" But I know my eyebrows must have reflexively furrowed, that my mouth was hanging open a little.

It was as though these women had become little green men, trying to convince me I was really going to enjoy my time on Mars. They seemed nice and well-meaning enough, but I wasn't buying a word of it.

Now I see we were just coming at summer from totally different vantage points.

Unlike them, I'd yet to experience head-banging homework battles or the violent cattle-prodding it takes to get to karate on time. All of that would come later (and with a *vengeance*). Only then would I come to better appreciate summer—or at least the promise of a few weeks off from scurrying/flailing/haranguing.

All I knew back then was that I was finally at a place where I could push a cart through the store without short grabby arms lurching for the Froot Loops. I'd discovered a whole new world, and I wanted to stay there.

Summer threatened to take it all away, exchanging my newfound freedom for the lie of "lazy days."

With little kids in the house, let's not kid ourselves. "Lazy days" are *hard work*. And here's just the short list of the tasks those "lazy days" might entail:

- Packing a phalanx of snacks and sippy cups;
- Forcibly applying sunscreen and bug spray to bodies bolting in the opposite direction;
- Hawkishly supervising all activities to ensure safety, minimize clothing ruination, and prevent sticks going into eyes;
- Hosing down muddy/sandy/screeching children;
- Prying off sopping wet clothing suctioned onto skin;
- Scraping residual mud and dung from the crevices of tiny sandals;
- Slapping together something that passes in some cultures as "lunch";

- Praying that at least one small person naps;
- Crumpling into a heap to puzzle over what we'll do post-nap and what to feed this crowd for dinner;
- Marking another day off the calendar until the glorious moment when school is back in session.

To live through a summer with little kids, I believe nothing short of an action hero is needed.

Yes, my friends, in the face of such challenges, a motherly MacGyver must rise up.

Because each new summer day will bring its own crisis. And in those weeks unaided by summer camp or Vacation Bible School, summer calls on moms everywhere to survive on their wits and the craftiest possible use of bubble solution, shaving cream, and a baby pool.

On *MacGyver*, something almost always blows up along the way. In the mom version, what's usually blowing up is our sanity. (Luckily, most of it grows back after the kids return to school. At least I *think* it does.)

Being a Mom MacGyver of Summer demands some hard-core survival strategies if we're to make it out alive. Thus, we scour parenting magazines. We "pin" our brains out. And we are rewarded with "1,001 Summer Fun Ideas!" (not one of which I actually want to do).

There's a whole cottage industry of folks, armed with glue guns and unquenchable zeal, who have become these Ambassadors of Summer Fun. It's their mission in life to show the huddled masses how you, too, can fill your children's every summer moment with rays of memory-making sunshine!

Nine out of ten Summer Fun Experts agree: You need a bucket. Next, you need to fill said bucket with Popsicle sticks that say cute things like, "Play bubble-wrap hopscotch," "Paint with pudding," or "Go geocaching." The idea is that your kids can delight in a new

"Boredom Buster!" every day, while you bask in the glow of your successful summer parenting.

In moments of pure desperation, I find myself skimming these lists for something, *anything*, that I wouldn't dread like the plague ... like painting with pudding. Bleck.

Call me crazy or call me lazy (I happen to be a little of both), but I don't *want* to make lava lamps or my own Play-Doh.

Okay, I'll just come right out and say it: *I want to do as little as possible*. Isn't that the whole point of summer—for kids to have at least one season of life to just be *bored* and figure it out?

The problem is that we modern parents fear boredom more than our kids do. We'll drag the brood from the mall to the movies to the monkey bars all day long rather than face the bickering, whining, and slumpy listlessness of boredom.

But I believe this with every fiber of my being: boredom does a body good.

And that's why—as my kids get old enough not to run around with plastic bags over their heads for more than a minute—I'm now easing *them* into MacGyver mode.

Now it's on *them* to take this magnifying glass, this roll of duct tape, and this tub of Legos and jury-rig something fun out of it—preferably something that does not explode. (They dare not pester me unless and until it does.)

I've done my time as a Mom MacGyver of Summer. So run along, kiddies. Go whip up your own fun and mayhem for a change.

This Mom MacGyver is long overdue for a nap.

How the Grinch Mom Stole Christmas

December 2013

Spoiler Alert: The following reveals certain covert operations at the North Pole and is not suitable for gullible children under the age of eleven. (In other words, hide this from your kids.)

I've had a decade to get my story straight. You'd think I'd have a plan by now.

It's no big surprise that nine-year-old Will has been peppering me with lots of "is Santa real" questions this year. It's become his annual tradition . . . as have my sweaty, shifty-eyed replies like, "What do *you* think?" and "Well, that's *ridiculous!*"

My muffed swings at all his questions seemed to work well enough before, mainly because the kid didn't *really* want to know. And because he was completely convinced we were too cheap and witless to pull off a decent Christmas without backup.

But this year, the questions have gotten deeper and harder to fake. He's been sending out stumpers like, "Why does Santa only give presents to rich kids and not poor kids around the world?"

I was pretty sure that calling Santa a racist one-percenter wasn't the jolliest course, so I came back at him with my most convincing blank stare.

The kid's been laying traps for me since Halloween—quizzing me with a side-eyed reporter's squint, trying to catch me in a jokey slip-up.

So by early December, when he asked me point blank, "Mommy, is Santa real?" I couldn't think of another angle to play. I cracked.

Looking back on it now, I wish I'd just sing-songed, "If you don't believe, Santa doesn't come! Tra la la!" Case closed. Magic preserved.

But instead, I decided to get all truthy with him, which was the absolute worst.

I sat him down quietly, looked deep into his huge Cindy Lou Who eyes, and I sighed. A lot. I mean, there was an excessive amount of sighing, followed by long stretches of helpless staring at the ceiling.

I gathered what few sweaty thoughts I had left and tried to string them together. Something about St. Nicholas being a real person who lived long ago and gave generously to children, who modeled kindness that we have tried to emulate for generations since. Something about the spirit of Christmas being very much alive.

When I finally shut up and wanted to die of a broken heart, I looked pleadingly into my son's soul. Had I just made a huge mistake? Would he survive this news?

He shrugged and said, "I don't believe that."

He then proceeded to jot out a brand new Santa letter, itemizing his top forty wish list items, and letting the fat man know there was a Home Depot nearby should the sleigh need repairs.

Okay . . . glad we had this talk.

Clearly I'd needed to do a little more research on how to create the perfect Santa let-down scene. I was convinced I had damaged Will's tender childlike wonder for all eternity.

But a couple weeks later, believe it or not, he came back for more. He told me he'd been discussing the matter with a buddy who'd recently joined the skeptic list, too. Will assured me he hadn't been the one to spill the beans, but together they had come to some manly conclusions about this whole Santa thing.

Will told me how he shared with his friend some weird rambling version of my Santa talk, something about an old guy "thousands" of years ago who gave "presents to the generations." I'm sure not one word of it made sense.

But sitting at his bedside that night, Will and I had the best conversation we've ever had—one where we giggled conspiratorially about all the times I'd screwed up playing the Tooth Fairy and other secret society things that were now revealed.

He got the joke now. And with a little sister left to fool, Christmas still felt merry—in a different, more knowing way, but with plenty of good stuff to spare.

As terrifically as I thought I'd screwed that whole thing up, it turns out I *wasn't* the Grinch who stole Christmas after all.

I *hadn't* stopped Christmas from coming. It came!

Someway or another, it came just the same.

(Even so, I definitely recommend lying. *Definitely.*)

Snow is a Four-Letter Word
February 2011

I still remember a time when nothing could stir my heart with gladness more than two little words: SNOW. DAY.

It was one of childhood's greatest joys—that out-of-nowhere, midwinter reprieve from pencils, books, and teacher's dirty looks.

There would be snow angels and cocoa with faux marshmallows and happy snowsuit romping 'til our frostbitten extremities fell off.

Like every kid who ever survived those days of unattended downhill sledding too close to car fenders and privet hedges, this was the stuff I lived for in the big, boring, middle of winter.

Today, I'm pretty sure all these blankety-blank snow days will be the slow and painful death of me.

The sound of my phone ringing at 5 a.m., the sight of the school name on my Caller ID, the very utterance of the words *snow day* makes every part of my face contort—jaws locked, lips pursed, nostrils flared, eyes rolled back in my head.

With the constant "wintry mix" onslaught of life in New England, my face could quite literally freeze this way.

Granted, I'm a Southern girl, and we embrace the white stuff in small doses . . . preferably in *centimeters*.

We think it's pretty for a while. We think it's fun to make that first (and hopefully last) snowman. Then we all agree: it needs to go away.

Even beyond my cultural limitations, I've got this pesky thing on my desk called a "calendar." It's filled with hilarious little words like "plans" and "deadlines" that don't go away no matter how much precipitation falls or how many children are suddenly underfoot.

So as much as I'd love to be that mom who smiles like a lunatic at the words *snow day* and whips out the cookie sheets, I'll admit it: I'm the grouchy mom who drags around the house in her bathrobe, muttering and shooting my kids the stink eye.

I'm starting to worry that the loony Ally Sheedy character from *The Breakfast Club* might be right. (Not about making snow with your own dandruff; we're all set, thanks.) But about that thing she said through tears and layers of heavy black eyeliner: "When you grow up, your heart dies."

It seemed a tad melodramatic at the time, but is that what's happened to me? Am I just a jaded old hag without a drop of childlike wonder left in me?

Because when I look out the window at a winter wonderland, I don't exactly whoop with joy; I sigh with pained inconvenience.

I don't dream of catching snowflakes on my tongue; I grouse about wet boots trudging all over my carpet.

I don't get out there and throw snowballs; I plunk the kids down in front of a screen.

I'm officially old. And a crank. And my feet are *never* not cold.

Somebody needs to launch into a pep talk—maybe one that says, "If life gives you lemons, make lemonade." Or to be more *au courant*, "If life gives you snow piles taller than your first-born, make snow cream."

That's what *my* mom did, and she probably got sick of snow days, too.

I guess we might as well do *something*. Lord knows we're stocked up on milk, and I have so many feelings that need eating.

That's How the Christmas Cookie Crumbles

December 2010

I remember one Christmas when my mother had it all together. Just *one.*

That one fine year, I'd come home from school most December afternoons and find something new under our tree, topped with a cheap stick-on bow. This level of advance preparation was something new and rare in our house, something peaceful and enchanting. I loved that year.

Every other Christmas of my memory involved Mom's traditional Christmas Eve scavenger hunt for the Lost Treasures of Yule. This was followed by the annual late-night wrapping frenzy of flying Scotch tape and dime-store paper.

My mom's holiday hurriedness would reach its crescendo on Christmas afternoon when she would let out a gasp, dash off to the underbelly of the spare bed, and unearth a tambourine or a latch hook kit she'd tucked away and forgot ever existed. (I wonder if that's where the Snoopy Sno-Cone Machine is that I never got . . .)

———————

As dearly as I'd hoped to usher in my own motherly Christmases all cool, calm, and curling-ribboned, history has a way of repeating itself.

Thirty years later, I find myself acting out updated (but somehow even more bedraggled) versions of this familiar holiday classic—like the day my daughter and I so thoughtfully brought cookies to the school bus driver.

I was commiserating at the bus stop with another mom friend, recounting all that was frazzling us in those blink-and-they're-done days till Christmas. She had a ticking time bomb of a sickly husband, ready to stick the stomach bug in everyone's stockings. I had all these wildly insurmountable work deadlines, stacked on top of my towering pile of unwritten Christmas cards. Neither of us had wrapped the first gift—cheapie bows or none. Together we threw aside *O Holy Night* and sang a rousing chorus of *O Holy Crap.*

On that day's to-do list, the single solitary item I'd checked off was one little bag of Christmas cookies for the bus driver. (Never mind that I'd cheated and bought them from the high school bake sale.)

Lucy wanted to present the cookies herself, which I told myself would be a lovely way for her to act out the spirit of giving . . . or some baloney like that. Why were my Spidey senses not tingling like mad as I placed this precious Christmas cargo into my daughter's wee hands?

Oh, you know what happened next.

Lucy heard the bus coming. She ran. She tripped. She fumbled the bag, which fell to Earth in a crumbly crash.

Even in their hard-knock condition, I still think those cookies would have passed inspection. (My seasonal standards were perilously low at this point.) But then my darling daughter—like Godzilla trudging through Tokyo—staggered, stumbled, and *stomped* all over my pretty bag of cookies.

There lay my one yuletide accomplishment in pieces on the ground, the bag busted wide, its sugary entrails sprinkled with grass and sand.

I suddenly morphed into Marlon Brando, hands on my head, crying heavenward in holiday agony, "LLLUUUUUCCCYYYYY!"

Then like some inept schlubby Magi, I toted my humble gift back home in defeat and added these words to my to-do list: *Get bus driver a Dunkin' Donuts gift card.*

The death of those cookies felt like the last holiday straw—as if some gnarly green fingers had come along and snatched my last can of Who Hash.

But after I stopped glowering and fuming, all I could do was double over and laugh.

As the story goes, my Grinchy heart grew three sizes that day. Because ready or not, perfect or not, Christmas was coming . . . and not from a store. (Or someone else's oven).

Christmas, I mused, must mean a little bit more.

Therefore, in the true spirit of the season, I did what had to be done. I smiled. I reflected on all my many blessings. Then I flicked the grass off those cookie shards and ate them for breakfast.

I'm sure it's what the bus driver would have wanted.

While Shepherds Walloped Their Flocks by Night

December 2011

I'm a bit shamefaced to report that Lucy chose to be "held back" in this year's church Christmas pageant.

After three good years running with the flock, our little lamb was supposed to trade in her furry ears and graduate to the big kid angel choir. Unfortunately, this was a promotion she wasn't remotely interested in pursuing.

I, of course, interpreted this commitment to the sheephood as a failure to embrace life's new challenges.

But who could really blame her? Sheep do have all the fun, frolicking on all fours, stealing the show right out from under the baby Jesus. All the angels do is sit primly in the choir loft, looking bored in their itchy tinsel halos.

All is calm. All is bright. All is zzzzz.

Big brother Will, meanwhile, was tasked with reprising his role of a seven-year-old shepherd, the toes of his white tube socks poking out from his leather fisherman's sandals.

Even though last year he'd bellowed with all the authority he could muster—"Let us go and see the child that the angels have told us about!" (or some such show of leadership)—this year Will begged off of doing any lines.

And by "begged off," I mean he just stared in silence at the pageant director when she asked if he'd take a speaking part, telepathically informing her that he wasn't so into it this year.

Again, I did not see this as progress.

But of course the moment my offspring took the stage, I forgot my hang-ups and videotaped my brains out.

It was clear from the start that this would be Lucy's Oscar moment, the last hurrah of a diva ready for her close-up. She threw herself completely into character.

From her fleecy ears and pinned-on tail down to her fake woolly Uggs, the girl looked the part. Her once-white shirtsleeves had turned brownish, stained with the chocolaty remains of Christmas candy that had recently gone in her mouth. Or near it.

Next to her motley crew of costars, Lucy's soiled white ensemble seemed the height of gritty realism. One fellow sheep sported the traditional furry ears and tail . . . and a crimson jumper dotted with Scottie dogs. Another rocked a sparkly purple *Flashdance* shirt emblazoned with a giant peace sign. My little lamb couldn't help but stand out in this distinctly un-Bethlehem-like menagerie.

Standing next to Lucy on stage was her shepherd brother, whose long fuzzy vest she began to paw at relentlessly like it was Lady Gaga's meat dress.

He valiantly tried to focus on the archangel's message of redemption for all mankind, but it was no use. The sheep pestered, pawed, and clamored for attention until, finally, he could stand it no more. In a flash of annoyance, Will turned to the little sheep at his feet and swept down his crook as if to wrangle her by the neck.

But just when you thought the tough guy shepherd was about to launch this sheep into the vestibule, his whole countenance changed. Instead of pounding her, he stooped gently to pet her little head.

Awwww. (That's what everyone in the pews said, anyway.)

Something about that scene rang true to me, as though this was their sibling relationship writ large on the stage. This is what their give-and-take usually looks like—a mutual peevishness that makes one want to clunk the other with a big stick—but underneath it all, there's a great big love. The kind they'd be lost without.

But even more than that, I couldn't help but think of another Shepherd and a certain ragtag sheep I happen to know. And I thought of all the times He's surely been tempted to wallop me, yet again and again, He chooses to simply love me.

Here was a scene of grace. Here was the message of Christmas— brought to you by my developmentally arrested children.

You're welcome. And Merry Christmas.

PART VII

SOAPBOX RANTS AND NEUROTIC HANDWRINGING

We've all got stuff that sends us into orbit.

You want the quickest way to launch me into "Aunt Linda" mode? (Kristen Wiig's eye-rolling *SNL* character is *me* right down to the turtle-neck.) Just start talking to me about screens and the comatose children who love them, this sex-drenched culture that won't leave our children alone for five whole minutes, and kale smoothies at school birthday par-ties. (Okay, that's not really a thing, but I bet *it will be.*)

This section has lots of words about the shorts-grinding stuff of life and motherhood that really sticks in my craw. But somehow this hand-ful of essays didn't seem to quite cover the full gamut of my crankiness.

So for reference, I've put together a quick list of things that I *didn't* rant about but *could have*—and I most definitely *will* if you bait me at a dinner party. Just be ready, because I have *thoughts*.

This list could have been titled, "First World Problems," but I believe that diminishes the *seriousness* of my thoughts on these pressing issues of today. Instead, I will call this list, "Stuff that Chaps My Hide."

It's my hope that this list chaps your hide, as well, so that we can be lifelong friends.

If you somehow don't share all my hide-chapping views, I'll still love you—even if you drink kale smoothies.

I think I will, anyway.

I mean, I'll try very hard.

Stuff that Chaps My Hide

1. Pet owners who call their dogs "fur babies" and/or plaster their Prius with paw-shaped magnets that say things like, "My grandchild is a Labradoodle."
2. Bluetooth talkers. First you think they're certifiably insane, then you realize they're just obnoxious. I'm not sure which is worse.
3. Blue raspberry-flavored *anything*. A blue raspberry does not exist in nature, thus it is clearly not God's will for His people.
4. Cryptic pity-seeking social media posts like "Unspoken prayer request!" or "My heart is breaking" or my personal favorite, a map pointing to the Emergency Room. This apparently chaps so many hides that it's earned the term *vaguebooking*, which makes my hide happy again.
5. #blessed.
6. The retina-burning color palette of a Justice store.
7. The olfactory-burning sensation of walking by—just walking by!—a Yankee Candle store.
8. People who take themselves way too seriously at karaoke, as if their inner Mariah is going to get "discovered" at some dive bar in Myrtle Beach.
9. Non-celiacs who order everything gluten-free for some nonsensical, trendy reason. Bread is life.
10. Grown men who wear Crocs. I'm pretty sure this isn't still going on, and for good reason—they've moved on to man buns.
11. One-ply toilet paper. (This *literally* chaps my hide.)
12. "Nontraditional" baby name spellings. I shouldn't give examples since one of them might be *your* kid's name, and that would be *awkward*. But let's just say, if you traded in the "y" on the end for an "i"—or if you just went way overboard with a cluster of unnecessary vowels—that's rarely a wise long-term career move for your child. I say, stick with what works. Which isn't Khaeitlynne.
13. Selfie sticks.

14. That thing Millennials do where they end every sentence with a Valley Girl-ish question mark? When I hear actual Ivy Leaguers talking this way on NPR of all places, I weep for the future.
15. I also really hate vacuuming carpeted stairs. It's *hard*, y'all.
16. When you call customer service, and you get their wretched voice recognition system because apparently no actual human beings work there *anywhere*. Nothing makes me want to end it all like hearing a Eurotrash robot coo, "I'm sorry, but I do not recognize your request." *Perhaps* my request wasn't *recognized* because it was peppered with such a dazzling array of expletives. (I've been known to save them up for special occasions.)
17. Geez, I sure have a lot of these. I may actually need to talk to a professional. But wait, *I have more.*
18. Drivers who ride their brakes going uphill. I'm not even sure how this is possible.
19. One-uppers who never let you finish a sentence.
20. Dog treat bakeries.
21. *I can keep going!*
22. Couple shoppers at the grocery store who stand there all day, analyzing the yogurt flavors together!
23. The wacko new way they're teaching kids math!
24. The phrase *Just sayin'!*

Okay, I'm really sorry. This is getting out of control.

I'm turning into Animal, just beating my poor drum set to a pulp. Next thing you know, I'll be collapsed in a heap, panting and fluttering my exhausted eyelids. Ranting sure can take it out of a person.

But wait, how did we not talk about tofurky?

Or that pizza crust that's stuffed with even *more* cheese?

Or the sacrilege of blueberry-flavored coffee?

Seriously, I'm done. I'm going to my happy place now. I'm totally zen, I swear.

Until someone brings up those whiny couples on *Property Brothers*. Then it's *on*.

Southern Discomfort: One Southerner's Struggle to Raise Decent, God-Fearing Children North of the Mason-Dixon

January 2009

"That's the first time I ever heard of a Yankee doing a decent thing," said Grandma, as if she regretted hearing anything good about the invaders."
—*Margaret Mitchell,* Gone with the Wind

I never thought I'd see the day. I am the mother of Yankee children.

Lucy is one of *them*—the product of a dyed-in-the-wool Carolina mother and a moved-around-a-good-bit Midwestern father raising their kids in New England. At three years old, she's finding her little voice now, which unfortunately sounds a lot like a Connecticut shipyard worker (minus the cursing).

While I try to approach the English language with the gentle lilt of Scarlett O'Hara or at least the good-natured twang of Elly May Clampett, my daughter sounds more like a miniature Fran Drescher.

The word *car* out of Lucy's lips mysteriously sounds like "koi." *Airport* becomes "airpoit." Even worse, the child has no idea what a collard green is. (Maybe you don't either. But trust me, it's a problem.)

I feel like I'm failing as a mother—at least as a *Southern* mother raising her brood in exile.

When my husband and I moved to Connecticut eight years ago, we embraced the newness of it all like foreign exchange students in a far-away land. Our friends and family humored our decision as best they could—until we announced the pending arrival of our first child. One South Carolina friend asked me in all seriousness, "So are you going to have the baby up there? Or are you going to come down here to have it?"

The very idea of bringing a child into this world anywhere but the South was clearly an abomination.

It was fine to go off and have our fun for a while, but it was expected that, at some point, we'd come to our senses and come home. How else could we raise this child right?

I've wondered that myself.

How will my kids ever know the messy glory of a pig-picking or the taste sensation of sweet tea? How will their ears thrill to the twangy beauty of mountain music? How am I supposed to pass on some great Southern legacy when every time I try to make biscuits, I end up screaming at the globby mess on my rolling pin?

It won't be easy.

We have dear friends here who are a bi-regional couple—Alaine from New Jersey and Scott from the Florida panhandle (probably the only legitimately Southern part of the whole state). When their daughter was born, Scott touched her feet to a handful of red clay he'd collected from home—just so the first earth touching her toes would be Southern soil.

Still, that little girl can't help but be a product of her environment. When she'd play with the kitschy Civil War action figures they bought her, her favorite general was—you guessed it—Ulysses S. Grant. This is what we're up against.

Most days, I love life in New England—especially on those not-so-frigid days when I get to eat real pizza and look out my window at a scene fit for a postcard. There's a lot to love.

But there's a lot I miss about the South that I worry my children will never know. Like the South's crazy cast of characters, like people who wave at you for no good reason, like not being in the minority when you say you go to church, like bluegrass, boiled peanuts, and colorful turns of phrase like *Ain't seen y'all in a coon's age.*

From a thousand miles away, I want my children to love what will seem to them like an exotic, faraway land.

Pat Conroy's mother used to read *Gone with the Wind* to him as a child so he could appreciate the honor, drama, and that hint of madness lying deep within his Southern roots.

I'm just wondering, is three years old too young to start?

Let's Have a Moment of Silence for the Cupcake

October 2008

Darkness has fallen upon the playground. Birthday cupcakes have been banned at my son's preschool.

All my life I've waited for the day when I could be the one to bear the Tupperware container of love, spreading joy and frosting to all my kid's little friends.

Mine was a summer birthday, so we few unfortunate July babies got cut out of the cupcake scene altogether. I remember gazing wistfully at my classmates being feted with sugar bombs—and I waited.

I waited decades upon decades until I birthed Willis one February and Lucy another November—and even longer till the moment I could make my own child the class hero for the day with my glad sugary tidings.

I never knew I'd only have one shot before they took it all away.

My one moment in the sun came during Will's first year of pre-school. It felt like I'd completed the journey to Real Motherhood. I sailed around the classroom on angel wings, stooping low to share my cupcake bounty and my Thomas the Tank Engine napkins, trying not to cry at the sight of three-year-olds singing to my little boy in the construction paper crown.

It was to be my first and last school cupcake party—despite my worthless investment in that beautiful new $20 cupcake caddy.

So I guess this year I'll have to come up with something more in keeping with the school's goal of "healthy choices"—perhaps some fruity kabobs or sawdust-laden bran muffins. Because nothing says "Have the Best Birthday Ever" like a celery stick slathered with peanut butter. (Come to think of it, the school's also nut-free—so let's just strip that stalk bare and call it a day.)

All I can say is—and I mean this with all due respect—*what a bunch of party poopers.*

I'm guessing whoever came up with this new rule is the same crowd doling out toothbrushes on Halloween. It's anathema, people. It goes against all we stand for in this country—like life, liberty, the pursuit of happiness, and a little thing we like to call *apple pie.*

I don't have anything against health. I could use more of it. And of course, cupcakes have their perils. (The ones with the bright blue icing will make your child poop the most brilliant shade of indigo. You've been warned.)

All I'm saying is, in the blink of the eye that is childhood, my kid was supposed to get five minutes per year to wear a silly hat and smear his face with sprinkles and be the Chosen One. Five minutes. That's all I was asking for.

Because before long, sprinkles won't be enough. He'll want a car.

So let us bid a fond farewell to "school birthday cupcakes" as they join the growing list of simple pleasures of youth now forbidden. (Remember licking the beaters and riding your bike without a helmet and playing with tiny balls of mercury? Okay, that mercury thing really was bad. But you get what I'm saying.)

Yet another childhood joy bites the dust.

Which, I might add, is exactly what those birthday graham crackers will taste like.

Freedom is Just Another Word for "Get Out and Stay Out"
August 2011

Many moons ago, in the faded mist of my childhood, there stood a corner grocery. It waited expectantly just down the hill from my small-town split-level. On summer afternoons when there was a lull in the day's exploring, a neighbor girl and I would bebop our way down the hill in search of jawbreakers or Pixy Stix.

We did this at the tender age of six.

We did this without Mom or minivan.

We did this with no one watching or caring.

We did this at least once without money (followed by a forced march back to apologize and cough up the cash for that lifted fistful of Atomic Fireballs).

I'm pretty sure this never happens now (I mean, the part about little kids going to the store unaccompanied ... not the shoplifting part).

Let me state for the record: you couldn't meet a less adventurous spirit than me. If there was the remotest threat of abrasion, water going up my nose, or adult displeasure, I was off the case.

Yet my tamest youthful exploits still manage to make my kids look like *The Boy in the Plastic Bubble*.

I skated straight down hills without padding. I bounced around the flatbed of a moving pickup without being strapped to anything. I explored poison ivy–infested woods without leaving a trail of text message breadcrumbs.

My childhood wasn't exactly a *Jackass* episode; I was just goofing around, usually without anybody paying much attention.

Come to think of it, I don't recall my mother being anywhere nearby in these scenarios. Grown-ups were rightly off doing the boring stuff that grown-ups do. Still, I knew she was on hot standby with a kiss and that god-awful Mercurochrome when a skinned knee called for it.

People say it's a different world now, and maybe it is. Or maybe we've watched one too many episodes of *To Catch a Predator*.

But remembering how children once happily roamed their little worlds from dawn till dinner bell, and knowing that most children don't have that chance anymore, makes me sad. And it makes me wonder: when our kids can't figure out how to just go out and *play*, have we done this to ourselves?

When my first and second grader can't contain themselves from coming in and out all day, bugging me for snacks, wanting to know where their Nerf pellets are, wondering aloud and with deep sighing what they should do next (while leaving the front door wide open with the air-conditioning on), I wonder.

Have we brought on this misery by not just kicking our kids out and locking the door? (A friend's mom reportedly used to do this, and by golly, I say it's an idea whose time has come again.)

When we shuttle our kids all over God's green Earth all the livelong day, are we raising kids who aren't bored long enough to think their way out of a recyclable shopping bag?

When we park ourselves in a nearby lawn chair and cluck, "Careful, honey!" over every misstep, are we training kids to think they need us—even when they really don't?

Are we the reason our kids refuse to leave the grown-ups alone to chat? Because we never seem to leave *them* alone either?

I'm just as scared as anybody of sex offenders, broken limbs, falling anvils, etc. By the same token, when I get daring enough to let my kids go to the playground one street over without me, then it's time to be scared someone will call me a bad mother (or worse, call Child Protective Services).

But honest and true, what ought to scare us most is that we'll raise kids with no imagination, no independence, no capacity for life, and (most terrifying of all) no plans to ever leave the house.

So what's a modern mother to do?

I suppose the first tastes of freedom have to come in bite-sized bits—letting the leash out a little further (figuratively speaking, of course; I've already shared my snarky views on baby leashes), letting them stay bored a little longer, slamming the door behind them a little harder.

Oh yeah, and locking it.

At least long enough to go to the bathroom all by myself.

The Face
September 2008

Will just gave me The Face.

The Face is my four-year-old's go-to look of displeasure—the one with the *Calvin and Hobbes*–esque nose crinkle, knit brows, and wildly protruding lips. It screams silently (when not accompanied by an *actual* scream) that he has suffered a grave injustice that must be protested.

He uses The Face a lot.

Like just now. I was naive enough to think the kid was napping. Then I heard the ear-splitting screech of his recorder emanating from the bedroom—the *same* bedroom where his baby sister was *sleeping*.

Enter me—great motherly killjoy—bounding through the door and hissing that I shouldn't have to *explain* why you don't go around clanging cymbals by your sleeping sister's bedside. In mid-screech, I grabbed the recorder. Cue The Face. (You can't miss it. It's frozen that way.)

The Face makes the perfect companion piece for timeless retorts like "Okay, okay, okaaaaay!" or "I'm mad at you!" or the fall-back "It's not fair!" Will's personal favorite is the ever reasonable "Just let me do what *I* want to do!" (e.g., bite my toenails at the dinner table or drink my own bath water or mash neon green Silly Putty into the carpet). This is just a sampling of the productive endeavors I have prevented him from pursuing.

I am indeed a hideous ogre.

On rare occasions, I see his point, like when I'm making him share (everybody hates that) or eat something greenish. I get it.

But day after day, Will goes to battle stations over things that just don't make a lick of sense to me. During lunch last week, for example, Will was good enough to retrieve his spoon from the floor. He did so, however—not with his hands, as is customary—but with the grimy grip of his outspread monkey toes.

When I dared insist that he get a clean spoon—one unsullied by toe jam—you would have thought I'd asked him to renounce God and country. He out and out refused, all the while giving me The Face—which led to a bad scene of time-outs, tantrums, and tufts of my hair being tugged out. All because he couldn't part with a crusty old foot-smudged spoon. It takes a village to figure kids out.

I know deep down that Will's just doing what kids do—testing the lines and seeing what happens when he crosses them, playing chicken with the Mack Truck that is Mom.

But too many times I've watched myself surrender the grown-up high ground, haranguing, fuming, and exploding into the childish hot-head I don't want my little boy to become.

Why do I always take The Face personally? I should just deal with such infractions like a traffic cop (preferably one in mirrored shades to hide the flames shooting from his eyes). Cool as a cucumber, that guy just strolls up with his notepad and jots out tickets for bad behavior—without waffling, squabbling, or making a big stink out of it.

That's my new goal—to show up to the scene of The Face like an über-cool Robocop Mom and dole out swift justice (minus the R-rated language and violence).

But if stuff goes sideways—escalating to "washing your mouth out with soap" proportions—let the record show that I've got an arsenal of Ivory at home, and I'm not afraid to use it.

Mastering the Machete
in a Silver Spoon World
October 2012

A little girl from the Amazon has taken up residence in my head.

I swear this never happens, but I just read an article in The *New Yorker* about a UCLA anthropologist traveling with an Amazon tribe. And as they were prepping for a leaf-gathering expedition down the Urubamba River, a little girl who was friends with the tribe asked if she could tag along. (Things must have been slow in the rain forest that day; maybe the cable was out.)

Now, correct me if I'm wrong, but if anybody in modern America got asked to bring along a random kid on a business trip, we'd all know it was a whiny disaster waiting to happen. We'd roll our eyes and stock the carry-on bag with every electronic diversionary tactic imaginable.

But this kid wasn't like most of *our* kids. This kid kept doing odd stuff. Like *helping*. This kid would sweep the entire tribe's sleeping mats not once, but twice, a day. She'd go fishing for crustaceans, which she'd clean (ewww), boil (presumably over hot, skin-melting flames), and serve the tribe for dinner—without ever being asked.

This kid was six years old. *Six.* My head can't quite process this information. *I* have a six-year-old girl, and I don't let her so much as stand in front of the microwave, much less boil up a lobster dinner.

So let me get this straight. You mean to tell me a six-year-old is capable of more than littering the house with all her Littlest Pet Shop crap, being shuttled around from play-dates to soccer practice, and dawdling? This *is* news.

That same anthropologist got involved in another study back home, this time examining middle-class families in Los Angeles. I've watched my share of *Beverly Hills 90210*, so it was no big shock to learn that the L.A. kids didn't lift the first entitled finger to nuke a Hot Pocket. The little girl with the fish-cleaning skills forced a question in the anthropologist's mind: why are these Third World children so darn useful to society and—I'm paraphrasing here—why do American kids do jack-squat?

Most of us stateside parents go around telling the same tired tale of woe—that if we dare ask a child to take a break from Angry Bird launching and take out the trash, there's such a lengthy appeals process you'd think they were being sent to the electric chair.

The *New Yorker* said this, not me: "Contemporary American kids may represent the most indulged young people in the history of the world." Ouch. Our kids are not just born with a silver spoon, but with a full-time staff of maids, chauffeurs, and bum-wipers whose *raison d'etre* is to make life "better" for their kids. Instead of giving children a leg up, the article wondered, are we crippling them by letting the muscles they need to make it through life just waste away?

Besides that, when a kid's life is focused on nothing more than the report card and the lacrosse field rather than adding value to their family and the world, aren't we dooming them to miss the point? To, in fact, feel a little pointless? Sheesh. Now that little Amazon girl is in my head. I see her there stoking the fire, wielding her machete with Julia Child–like finesse, and I'm forced to admit—my kids are capable of so much more than an Easy-Bake Oven. Nobody's saying Lucy should tend a vat of boiling oil. But the child could make her bed (if she could find it under all the mounds of stuffed animals). She could put away her laundry. Will could cut his own meat. He could make a few passes with the Hoover.

Hey, it could happen. It *should* happen.

Somebody needs to vacuum around here. And from the looks of this place, it ain't gonna be me.

Mom versus the Machine

Author's Note from The Future: This column was originally written in January 2011. Please forgive the use of archaic terms like VCR, which refers to a contraption from olden days that recorded TV shows on videotape (rather than a puffy cloud of Interweb air). I'm also not sure if kids still play with the DS thingees referred to here. If it helps you, Modern Mom of the Twenty-First Century, just substitute the word "phone" for "DS" in all references, and you're there.

If happiness is a warm puppy, then sadness is a cold, lonely bus seat.

Will rode home alone on the bus yesterday. Meanwhile, his first-grade buddies bunched up three to a bench with the new guy—a rude, unfeeling little lout named DS.

Nintendo DS.

For the uninitiated (and I include myself in that lot), the DS is this itty-bitty computer game gadget that appeared under most elementary schoolers' trees this Christmas and was met with squeals of delight (followed by hours of dead silence).

Ever since that infernal machine started making the daily trek to school with one of Will's friends, every boy in a three-bench radius seems to have fallen under its spell. Will used to cram his backpack full of Lego catalogs, ready to pore over every detail with a bus buddy and plan their next Lego war. But that's old news.

"All anybody wants to do is look at that DS," Will cried, his giant puppy-dog eyes filling with tears. "Nobody talks to me."

Okay, I'm a mother. You'll forgive me if I declare here and now: I hate those things.

I know it's painfully old-fashioned, but I don't think I'm alone. I want my kids to imagine great things in brains not yet turned to mush. I want my kids to run around and breathe outdoor oxygen. I want my kids to read actual books. I want my kids to talk to me and their friends instead of drooling over some screen.

And I don't want them to do what I did (and didn't do) when my parents finally gave in thirty or so Christmases ago and splurged on an Atari.

I did not perfect my backhand or practice piano—skills that would actually be useful in life. Instead, I played *Pitfall* for hours, perfecting the timing of how to spring across a series of bit-mapped crocodile snouts without becoming lunch.

I did not interact with my family. Sometimes I even played *Pac Man* right through dinner ("But I've got the high score!"), giving me the perfect escape into a place where my parents had no desire to follow.

I did not play outside with friends. We'd blow through whole sunny afternoons playing *Defender*. (Correction: My friend, Kate, played *Defender*. I'd get blasted out the sky after thirty seconds then glaze over while she showed off her freakish intergalactic warfare skills for the next hour.)

None of this was a huge deal. But man, was it ever a huge waste of time.

So here I am in the here and now, straddling this line where on one side I've got to stay tech-savvy enough to know the world my kids are inhabiting and the language they're speaking. It won't cut it to remain a clueless old bat who never learned to set the VCR while her kids are out teleporting to other dimensions.

But on the other side of that line, I'm also the parent. And if something tells me not to let the cyber-horse out of the barn just yet, I don't have to—no matter how much pressure builds that "everybody else" has smartphones, laptops, and their own Sims family.

I loved *Toy Story 3* (although Woody and the gang nearly being burned alive didn't go over well with my kiddos; they refuse to watch it ever again). In one review I read, the critic described the toys as "fighting for the right to be playthings again—for the sacred, make-believe pleasures of analog imagination that have been chased out of childhood by technology."

That sounds a lot like me at the moment—fighting for my children to live a while longer in a tech-free zone of innocence, ratty-haired dolls, and stuffed dogs with their noses loved off.

I'm going to cling to that ideal a little while longer, even if I know it can't last for infinity and beyond.

PART VIII

LIGHTNING BOLTS AND LIGHTBULB MOMENTS

Moments of epiphany come in many forms: an apple beaning Newton in the head. A blinding light on the road to Damascus. The moment Jay-Z met Beyoncé.

And I'd say those moments have yielded some pretty earth-shattering results: the discovery of gravity. The penning of the New Testament. *Crazy in Love* and Blue Ivy.

As epiphanies go, mine don't even come close. (They've never once led to a scientific discovery or a bootylicious jam.)

But I still try to find those "aha" moments whenever I can—while typing away from this cluttered, dusty, lonely desk. I stole this idea from Joan Didion, but it's 100-percent true: writing is how I figure out what I think.

And sometimes what I think is *way deep*. (You should see my musings on the works of Plato . . . I mean, *Dana* Plato.)

And sometimes what I think is woefully shallow. (I have spent an inordinate amount of time noodling over celebrity baby names.)

Either way, it's only when I put pen to paper that I'm able to put life's puzzle pieces together, glimpse the bigger picture, and make some sense of it all. (Except for that business of naming your kid North West. No one can make sense out of *that*.)

This section represents those rare moments of departure when I took it down a notch, struck my best Thinker pose, and got my ponder on.

So hike up those pant legs. It's about to get *deep* in here.

The Dark Side of the Balloon
October 2010

"Nobody can be uncheered with a balloon," says Pooh.

And while I usually consider the Bear of Little Brain the bastion of all wisdom, I have to take issue with him here.

As a mother (and this sounds heartless, so I'll just spit it out), I have come to *hate* balloons. If you ask me, they're nothing but bouncy balls of bliss one minute, instruments of torture the next.

Should you hand my child one of these nefarious "gifts," I will beam as though this is the most glorious day in human history. But inside, I'll be steeling myself for helium-induced heartache. Because we mothers know that after this ebullient (and all too brief) honeymoon period, there's nothing but a handful of unhappy eventualities left to us.

The same balloon that is now holding aloft all my child's hopes and dreams will either a) burst in his face, b) fly into the stratosphere, or c) be dead by morning. All of the above end in piteous sobs I'd just as soon avoid.

And don't even get me started on balloon animals.

Will's first balloon animal encounter was at my husband's company picnic. Shaped like a submarine he could wear as a hat, that thing was the highlight of his six-year-old life.

It really *was* ingenious, and I have to give props to those balloon-animal guys, gnarling their fingers into arthritic nubs after transforming balloons into pirate swords and butterflies for seven hours straight.

But telling Will that his prized inflatable hat would be shrunken down to a shriveled tube of latex within twenty-four hours—essentially that the spell would be broken by midnight and all would be as it was before—was like telling him there was no Santa Claus.

Then there was Lucy, who within nanoseconds of receiving her balloon dachshund was mourning the loss of her doggie's front leg, shivved by a blade of grass.

Even after six years of popping/flying/shriveling balloon experience, there was just no explaining to these children that balloons don't last forever, that we are brightened by them for a few days (or a few seconds) and then we move on.

When it came to this new, unimaginable wonder of balloon animals, none of that computed. Who could possibly be expected to part with their newfound treasures so painfully soon?

———

Despite the flood of cruel tears that have been wrought by these latex tormenters, I suppose I should be glad for the life lessons of the balloon.

My children don't know it yet, but the road ahead will be bumpy with the jolts of beloved things leaving us, either in the shock of a thunderbolt or with the slow hiss of loss.

Such inconsequential "starter sadnesses" as the balloon brings are life's training sessions—a bracing of the spine, a strengthening of the heart—for sadnesses to come that *do* matter.

This process of reaching out to take hold of some fragile joy (knowing it may not last and it may even bring sorrow) is all part of a life fully lived—maybe even the very best part.

So as much as I want to stand between my children and all of life's popping balloons, even *I* have to admit, it is far better to have loved a balloon and lost than never to have loved at all.

Little Kids and the Laws of Nature

February 2009

I'm not a science whiz, but I do know that certain laws of nature are set in stone.

What goes up must come down.

For every action, there is an equal and opposite reaction.

As temperature approaches absolute zero, the entropy of a system approaches a constant minimum. (Okay, I got that one off the Internet.)

After a few years in the parenting business, I'm also seeing some irrefutable laws of kiddie nature revealing themselves in this Petri dish of family life.

(I haven't sought formal approval of these theories from the guys in the white coats, but if you've got kids, I'm betting you can back me up.)

Law #1:

In the event that a mother should answer a ringing telephone, an otherwise happily-occupied child will be beset by the most urgent calamities—usually dire thirst, an inability to locate a missing Polly Pocket shoe, or an outburst of violence against another previously contented sibling.

When such needs are ignored, the volume of the child's request will increase until a response of equal or increased volume is returned (while one hand muffles the receiver) or until the child is redirected to an illuminated screen. (A similar phenomenon is experienced whenever a mother shuts a bathroom door or steps into a running shower.)

Law #2:

The natural resting state for a child's sippy cup in a mother's purse is upside down and dripping.

Law #3:

Male children are incapable of following the direction of a pointing finger. When a male child is directed toward a missing item of interest (usually located within a twelve-inch radius), he will look in all other possible directions (primarily skyward). The parent is then forced to enter the child's circumference, retrieve the desired item, and dangle it in front of the child before the object is discovered to loud exclamations of "I found it!"

Law #4:

The sight of a plate of food arriving piping hot from a restaurant kitchen is a psychological prompt for one or more young children to urgently require bathroom assistance.

Law #5:

A child who is spreading happiness by giggling and skipping through the living room will invariably make unhappy contact with a protruding coffee table corner.

Law #6:

When a parent expresses interest in viewing an adult television program (e.g., the nightly news), a child will immediately begin emitting a loud and nonsensical barrage of words, knock-knock jokes, or songs of his/her own composition until the program pauses for commercial. Immediately, said child will lapse into a trance-like state and exhibit symptoms of hypnosis at the sight of two old ladies doing tai chi in a public park. Once adult programming has resumed, the utterance of phrases such as *Gaza Strip* or *Dow Jones* will revive the entranced child and reignite vigorous chatter.

Law #7:

The aforementioned laws are inherent in the untamed mess of life with kids.

Law #8:

While it may go against all scientific reason, logic, and good sense, we can't help it: we love them to the nth degree anyway.

On the Ride of Our Lives—Without Training Wheels

April 2011

Here's a story with a *Don Quixote*–like impossible dream, a complicated hero who vanquishes his demons, and one of those heart-in-
your-throat endings worthy of Kerri Strug.

Will learned to ride a bike.

Okay, I know that sounds like teeny-tiny small potatoes, but trust
me. This is *Hallelujah Chorus*–worthy.

Will is seven, and he's had this shiny red bike that's the stuff of little
boy dreams since he turned four. Instead of being his greatest source
of boyhood joy, the bike has been his nemesis. He has feared it. He
has shirked from its very presence. He has thought up every excuse
imaginable not to go near it.

Bike-riding attempts have become nothing but a teary death
march for the boy, and a head-banger of an afternoon for his poor,
demoralized father. Glum and braced for failure, he'd creep along at
a snail's pace, tottering back and forth from one training wheel to
the other, certain he would keel over at any moment and turn into a
full-body scab.

It seemed a very real possibility that our child might be the first in
modern history to never learn to ride a bike.

Then a friend let me in on a hot tip that worked on her kid, one
I'm happy to share now with any other closeted parents of non-bikers
out there.

Here's what you do. Ditch those stupid training wheels. Then go
a radical step further and take off the pedals too. It sounds crazy, but
once Will got the feel for the balance of the beast (instead of leaning

on his training wheels like wobbly crutches), he was in the zone for the first time. (See? This crap *is* educational.)

Dad spent one Saturday pushing Will down our street pedal-free, giving him the chance to find his center, gain some confidence. Then the very next Saturday, the pedals went back on, Dad gave him one last fateful shove, and Will was soaring.

He was *actually* doing it. *Riding a bike.* Just like in the movie reel that plays in every parent's memory and will now always play in mine.

Better yet, he was riding like a wild man—turning, and swerving, and pretending to pop wheelies. Once, he even threw a jubilant fist into the air like a miniature Judd Nelson who'd just become part of "the club." I was beside myself.

Proud is way too small a word for what I was feeling. *About to wet my pants with joy* gets closer, but not quite.

Witnesses at the scene may have even caught me *skipping*.

You want to know the weirdest part? The very next weekend, this same kid who was whizzing by me with flames shooting off the handlebars would end up flat on his back in a hospital bed for two nights; his sickly, asthmatic, Evel Knievel lungs struggling for air. Future bike-riding exultation would have to wait.

But I guess parenting is like that.

It's that proverbial roller-coaster ride that one minute has you whooping it up and catching bugs in your big goofy grin, the next minute your hair's standing on end and everything's upside down. And occasionally, somebody pukes.

Now that we're back from our hospital adventure, I'm just trying to let that dizzy spell pass and get my legs back underneath me. I still feel a bit wobbly.

But no matter what corkscrew turns and death-defying loops are waiting around the bend (and there will be more I never even see coming), one thing's for sure: buying a ticket for this crazy ride was the best decision I ever made.

I'm pretty happy we kept the bike, too.

Breathe In, Breathe Out
April 2011

(Author's Note: Remember that hospital trip I just mentioned? Here's how that all went down.)

Well, that ambulance ride wasn't *at all* how I'd pictured it.

I thought I'd be huddling next to my child's gurney, clutching his hand like some TV movie guardian angel. Instead, I sat up front next to the burly EMT with pierced ears, staring dumbly out the window and wondering how the heck we ended up here.

It all started Thursday with a cough I didn't even notice.

By Friday, the cough had taken over Will's wheezy seven-year-old lungs, and those breathing treatments we pump into him when he's sick weren't making a dent. His belly was working overtime, up and down, in what seemed more like a ghoulish caricature of breathing than actual breathing.

We headed to the doctor, who sent us off with renewed hope that this prescription in my hand would do the trick. Instead, while we waited at the pharmacy counter, Will threw up in the nearest trashcan. And he threw up all night. And he kept breathing hard in and out. And nothing made it better.

I hated to make that 3 a.m. call to the pediatrician, afraid of what he might say.

He said it. He sent us into the dark of night to the emergency clinic, where they hooked up my wet noodle of a boy to IVs, pumped oxygen into his nose, and propped him up for X-rays, which revealed a hazy clump of pneumonia in his right lung.

Next thing you know, I'm watching the Saturday sunrise from an ambulance window en route to the hospital (the one part of this ordeal that Will now reports was "really fun").

The next two days in the hospital are a blur, probably because I could count on one hand the number of hours I'd slept in two nights. There was a lot of staring at ceiling tiles hand-painted by children who'd been patients in these rooms and a lot of staring at my little boy's tiny chest laboring to breathe.

The child looked like a refugee from a leper colony—all blotches and hives and tubes and far-away eyes. Will got so doped up overnight that when the nurse asked if he knew where he was, he mumbled, "Home."

As terrifying as it was to be there, I knew it *wasn't* home; it'd all be over soon. We'd do our time, they'd make him better, and we'd go back to our lives in a few days.

But for some folks on that pediatric ICU floor, I could see this place *had* become home. On visits to the communal family room, I'd smile at a mom throwing in a load of laundry, her hair wet from showering. This was her home for now.

We watched a young family—one of the children with a conspicuously bald head—gathering around a table of take-out sandwiches. This was their home for now.

We were the lucky ones. We'd be going home soon, a little shaken but stronger and ready to step right back into all of life's wonderful normalcy.

But all around us, families were there to stay—day after agonizing day, staring at those same ceiling tiles, praying, crying, and wondering what they'd have to go through to get their children back home again.

Mine was just the tiniest glimpse into a heartrending journey we thankfully have never had to walk. And I am grateful in a whole new way for the basic stuff of life—lungs that work, a home to go back to, undimmed hope for whatever comes next.

We are blessed. I never knew how blessed until now.

Truly, our cup—and sometimes even Will's gunky lungs—runneth over.

Paddle Your Kids!
(Oh, Wait . . . With . . . I Meant,
With Your Kids)

August 2008

No one could accuse me of being outdoorsy.

Sometimes I even bear a striking resemblance to Hayley Mills's evil stepmother-to-be in *The Parent Trap*, bursting out of her tent like Medusa in sponge curlers and shrieking, "Get me out of this stinkin' fresh air!"

It's not that I don't appreciate nature. I do. I just appreciate it best in perfect seventy-five-degree weather with zero humidity. Preferably from a hammock. Surrounded by a giant mosquito net.

That's why it surprises me that we have a canoe—and that I like it.

Every so often, all four of us pile in, each kid with his and her own cushion and mini-paddle. And we skim along the marshes, under railroad trestles, and over the swells of the Sound.

Even when there's whining, black flies, or both, it's a time that never fails to renew me somehow—maybe because it reminds me of all the great, big beauty in our world that I was *this* close to missing that day.

Because if it were up to me and Will (who shares my leanings against sweat and exertion), we'd all hole up at home and grow ever pastier.

But thankfully, Will has a father who itches to sweat and exert, and sometimes drags us along by the collective hair.

So we experience a world outside of our own—a world where we can spy on baby ospreys in their nests, paddle by craggy rocks dotted with sea birds, or spank jellyfish passers-by without mercy.

Then if we're lucky, we can stop off at some speck of an island, line up on a log of driftwood, and consume a tube of Pringles. For Will, that makes all the stinkin' fresh air worth breathing.

When I was a kid, the most back-to-nature thing my parents ever did with me was prod me into the garden to pick lima beans.

So if Will and Lucy can get past the bug bites and the soggy bottoms and the parents cranky from having to retrieve dropped paddles and abandoned flip-flops, this is the stuff of some seriously happy childhood memories.

It's not a bad deal for *me,* either. I can look out from my perch at the front of the canoe and be inspired by sights slightly more majestic than the towering laundry piles awaiting me back home.

And I need that—even if I usually have to be *reminded* that I need that.

Lucy (who is two and thus a seasoned expert in the subject of lackadaisical wandering) loves nothing better than cramming my nose into life's roses.

Take, for instance, our last canoe expedition. While everyone else was busy loading up after our Pringles pit stop, I watched Lucy wander over to a hill overlooking the cove and plop down.

There she sat, not digging in the muck, not collecting rusty nails or broken glass shards, just staring out at the water. It was that time of day when there's gold in the light.

"Whatcha doin'?" I asked her, a tad annoyed. (Couldn't she see this was no time for quiet reflection?)

Never looking up from her outward gaze, she simply and sweetly replied, "I lookin' to see what God made."

Oh.

So I dropped my stack of dripping life jackets and sat down beside her. And *I* looked, too.

Every now and then, it's awfully nice to put down the piles, take a look around, and be reminded.

And to think I was *this* close to missing it that day.

Two Sets of Feet on the Coffee Table, Four Little Hands to Hold

June 2008

A friend of ours died last week. Just forty years old with a wife and two little girls, he dropped dead in the garage. Nobody saw it coming.

I guess nobody ever really does. And that's the thought that's been needling at the back of my mind until it's now a forceful scratch, nudging me to appreciate the tangible truth of my husband's feet propped up on the coffee table next to mine. Or the sticky little hand tugging at my shirt.

When thoughts come of his wife, dumbstruck at becoming a widow, I can't help but think how blessed I am at this season, this unmarred season that is surely just that—a season. And when I remember her, I do what the clichés all say I'll do, and I squeeze my loved ones a little harder. I say "I love you" a little more often.

But then, to tell you the truth, I go about my business and forget. I get annoyed and bitter and bored and overwhelmed a thousand different ways each day, and I forget my fleeting moment of loving resolve.

In fact, I'll confess that from the moment I picked up my son from preschool today, the only thing I wanted to squeeze a little tighter was his scrawny little neck. The entire afternoon was nothing but one ungrateful whine after another.

The lollipop he'd chosen (and happily consumed) wasn't the flavor he'd *really* wanted. His sandwich was cut into the wrong shape. His juice wasn't drinkable without a bendable straw. His Popsicle was the wrong color. (I would like the record to show that none of the tyrant's demands were met.)

I wanted to hurl myself in front of a truck (or at least call shotgun) to save us both from another conversation about ingratitude and all the starving children in the world. If there was ever a day when I threw loving thoughts out the window, when I wanted to be anywhere but here, it was today.

And that's part of what bugged me so much. It made my head spin to see how quickly I could go from counting my blessings to keeping a record of wrongs. One minute, I'm vowing through tears to live in the moment. The next, I desperately want out of the moment.

I guess that's the great paradox of parenting—one minute it's maddening, the next it's magical. And sometimes the ratio of maddening to magical can be awfully lopsided.

But when I think of that young father leaving this world without warning, it's all too clear that even a lopsided day could—God forbid—be our last one together. So every now and then, I have to purposefully lift my head out of the choking weeds of the mundane, take a good look around my life, and remember what it's all for.

When a friend and I talked through the struggle that lies ahead for our mutual friend, she shared the words of someone she knew who'd lost her young daughter too soon.

"I played with my daughter every day, I prayed with her every day, I was there for her every day," that grieving mother had said. "I have no regrets."

There are no guarantees that two sets of feet will always rest upon our coffee table, that I'll always have these little hands in mine. One way or another, our time together will end. And when it does, I could ask for nothing more than to be able to say, "I have no regrets."

Speaking of which, there's a little boy playing at the train table who sure would be happy if I'd quit typing and join him.

That's an afternoon I'm not likely to regret anytime soon.

Driving and Crying
and Other Pastimes

Author's Note: When I wrote this essay, the words came pouring out like they had no other place to go—and so did the tears. I wrote this right after the Newtown, Connecticut, massacre in December 2012, when twenty precious little children were slain at school about an hour away from our door.

There is no funny here, so if you're in the mood for that right this minute, go read the one about mom jeans and come back to this later. Or better yet, go read David Sedaris. He's a sure thing.

I have all my best cries in the car. Only the eighteen-wheeler drivers see my pain, and that's the way I like it.

So as I drove to my children's school on that awful Friday afternoon, I clutched the wheel and sobbed like a baby.

It's okay. The president was crying, too. On the radio, I heard the leader of the free world choking on his words, as if he couldn't quite believe the horror of what he had to tell us.

In those five minutes of station wagon solitude I'd been given, I allowed myself to fall apart. There was ugly crying and wailing and maybe a little gnashing.

Then I did what I had to do—I put myself back together again.

And I did what twenty mothers and fathers in Newtown *couldn't* do—I picked up my children at elementary school.

My son and daughter took no notice of all the grim-faced grown-ups with red-rimmed eyes—or the knowing looks being exchanged above their heads. They wriggled against the strange new fervor in their mothers' hugs. They had no idea that the earth beneath our feet had shifted and shaken us hard that day.

All they knew was it was Friday, Christmas was coming, and all was right with the world. Which is just as it should be.

But ever since that day and all season long, I've been plagued by sneak attacks of sadness that my kids couldn't help but notice—like that time I crumpled into tears over a sink full of dishes. *O Holy Night* was playing on the radio, and those words of a weary world rejoicing rushed my heart and buckled my knees.

Then there was drop-off at school the Monday morning after, when I tried to act normal even as I gripped my bewildered children like a hungry boa constrictor. (There was, of course, more sobbing in the car all the way home. I'm now a pro at navigating with mascara runoff in my eyes.)

My children may also be wondering why I sometimes fix them with a look like I'm trying to memorize them—so I can remember just what it looks like to be seven years old, in that Santa hat with the jingle bell on it, singing that made-up song about loving me more than Christmas.

They don't know it, but I am burning their image to my hard drive. I am willing them never to change, to lose their innocence, to leave me here without them.

Our children thankfully appear to have no idea what's happened. I'm okay with that. I'm prepared to answer if they ask, but we have chosen not to tell them yet.

For now, anyway, we see no reason to fill their dreams—already too full of giant spiders and zombies—with murderous strangers. Please, not yet.

Of course, none of this was what anyone wanted. None of this can ever make sense or be made right.

The only thing that *did* make sense was the sunset we saw on the drive home from school that Friday.

What a black, broken day it had been. But there was that sunset, streaking over the waters of the Long Island Sound with every orange and pink God could think up. What an astoundingly beautiful place He intended this world to be. I'd forgotten.

Evil is certainly taking its toll, straining to reduce to ruins what the Maker meant for good.

But no matter how deep and close the shadows creep, a basic fact of life and physics holds true. In the battle of darkness and light, darkness loses. Every time.

I've never once opened a dark closet and watched the room go black. Instead, every single time I flick on the light, darkness runs for the corners—without fail.

Though we may have to wait a while to see it shining, the light always wins. *Always.*

So I will hold my candle a little higher than I did before this happened. I never realized before how badly we all need the light.

And I will go looking for sunsets. Because even if in my haze of sadness or busyness I miss the one God makes today, He's sure to paint another masterpiece tomorrow—*without fail.*

DEEDEE FILIATREAULT TRIES TO BE A FREELANCE WRITER WHILE HER KIDS (YADA YADA YADA . . .)

This goes out to my faithful, beloved readers who have followed this column from days gone by—way back when it appeared on actual newsprint that rubbed off on your fingers.

Back then, I ended every column with this little tagline: "DeeDee Filiatreault tries to be a freelance writer while her children _____." Then I'd fill in the blank with a wide selection of assorted mayhem.

I thought it'd be fun to compile those taglines all in one place, and it was. (For me, anyway.) Reading them now is like flipping through a box of old Polaroids, each snapshot filling in a story of childhood—and of a grown-up cobbling together her working life while that childhood happened.

Spoiler alert: Nowhere on this list do the words *quietly* or *help* appear.

This list transports me back in time—even while it reminds me that in our family (and probably yours, too), some things never, ever, *I mean ever* change.

Especially the "loud" and "not helping" parts.

DeeDee Filiatreault tries to be a freelance writer while her kids:

Argue over who won—at anything
Avoid their waterlogged sandbox full of spider eggs
Beg for blue yogurt in a tube
Beg for Doritos in their lunch boxes
Beg to watch videos
Belt made-up tunes in a glass-breaking falsetto
Belt out *Sweet House Alabama* (Yes, Lucy thinks it's "house")
Carpet the actual carpet with a gazillion Legos
Catch butterflies and doom them to a slow bughouse death
Chant "You've got to move it, move it!"
Collect nasty old seagull feathers in a jar
Come up with really bad knock-knock jokes
Congregate under her desk
Count every Nerd in a box of Halloween Nerds
Cut to shreds all those back-to-school catalogs
Dig up worms and try to make them pets
Do air guitar
Do battle with their battery-powered hamsters
"Do nothing" at school
Do science experiments with a Ken doll in the bathroom sink
Drop and give her twenty
Eat just the bunches from their Honey Bunches of Oats
Feed ants to the new "pet" praying mantis
Feign neglect and perfect the art of guilt trips
Gag on peas
Get sand in every imaginable crevice
Hang the fragile ornaments from the flimsy end of the branches
Invent new lyrics to "Grandma Got Run Over by a Reindeer"
Jump rope in the house
Lament the new "one-hour of screen time" resolution
Leave the caps off every marker in the box

Litter the floor with snotty tissues

Look on adoringly

Make a backyard fort out of sticks, stuffed animals, and a *Toy Story* umbrella

Make a super-spy platypus from Legos, complete with "evil eyebrow"

Make liquid soap "lemonade" in the sink

Make up Lego-themed lyrics to Mumford & Sons songs

Make up new excuses for not walking the dog they wanted

Nibble at stale peppermints glued to the gingerbread house

Paint their toenails with dry-erase markers

Peek under rocks in search of something gross

Perch stuffed animals on the ceiling fan blades

Perfect their pouting techniques

Pick fistfuls of plentiful dandelions from our yard

Pick gravel out of the neighbor's driveway for their rock collections

Pick out every pea that was snuck into the mac & cheese

Plot their alibis

Point out must-haves (like a penguin race track) in the latest toy catalog

Poke at fragile Christmas tree ornaments

Ponder the meaning of life

Pore over Halloween costume catalogs

Practice armpit farting like there's a scholarship to be won

Put on their swimsuits and pretend to be superheroes

Ram into the coffee table

"Read" *Entertainment Weekly* on the toilet

Refuse to eat turkey

Run the batteries down on everything in the house

Scatter Playmobil swords and hats for her vacuum to lunch upon

Scrounge for those fakey "fruit snacks"

Show her a flattened frog they just peeled off the road

Skewer each other with fishing poles

Sled down the stairs on pillows

Sneak cookies

Sneak extra toys into their backpacks

Stick address labels all over the craft table

Stomp ants in the driveway

Surprisingly develop calf muscles

Tape together garlands of yarn and cotton balls

Toil bitterly over their school valentines

Touch everything in sight with sticky candy cane hands

Trade Trash Packs like they're hog futures. (Don't know what Trash Packs are? Lucky you. I don't know what hog futures are, so we're even.)

Transform their room into a rain forest of typing paper vines and snakes

Try not to step on the tails of Lucy's invisible cats

Try out new material on their stuffed animals

Try out new ways of using *poop* in a sentence

Try to build a blanket fort over her desk

Try to smuggle Silly Bandz into their backpacks

Tug at her sleeve and say, "Excuse me, Mom" (over and over and over)

Turn every flat surface into a Lego table

Turn five minutes of homework into a half hour of harrumphing

Turn her old Fisher-Price castle into a Lego sniper nest

Unfortunately act their age

Walk around with oven mitts on their feet

Watch more than the recommended daily allowance of TV

Watch reruns of *The Andy Griffith Show*

Watch TV alongside a jar full of roly polies

Whack each other with Chinese yo-yos

Whack each other with leftover birthday balloons

Work on their Christmas lists (in October)

ACKNOWLEDGMENTS

I still have a Post-it somewhere with a chicken-scratch scribble that reads, "You've got a book in you, and it's gonna be good." Mark Chambers wrote that, the man who hired me for my first job as a real writer and, in so doing, completely shot off course the whole trajectory of my life. Thank you, Mark, wherever you are, for pushing me headlong into a career I never would have been brave enough to try. Thank you for poring over every word of every speech I ever wrote, telling me straight up (usually through a fog of cigar smoke) which words stunk and which ones sung. Your faith in me changed everything. I hope I've finally reached "Most Distinguished Ho" status in your eyes.

This book would never have seen the light of day if it weren't for Jen McMahon's big mouth. I can't thank you enough for your cheerleading, my crazy "red-headed" friend. And a million extra thanks to Holly Rubino at Skyhorse Publishing, who took over Jen's duties as cheer captain and really got this ball rolling. I miss our chats about Benedict Cumberbatch. Nicole Frail, you inherited me and my little book, and you have proven to be a most patient, skillful, and generous editor. I'll always be most grateful to *The (New London, CT) Day* newspaper, especially then-editor of *The Lyme Times*, Marisa Nadolney. I wrote her an email out of the clear blue 2007 sky that said, "How 'bout letting me write a humor column on parenting?" And she wrote back the unthinkable. She said, "Yes." I'm so thankful for all my faithful readers—both friends and strangers—that I've been blessed to gather up and take with me down this meandering road since that day.

I have strict criteria in choosing friends for life: they have to make me laugh. *Hard.* And oh, how I adore my funny band of friends—including (but *definitely* not limited to) Pam Lyon, Kendall Love, Scott Padgett, Susan Boffoli, Shannon Moody, Kate Bartlett, and all my Harlequin Honeys. Just trying to keep up with you has made me funnier—and my life richer. And of course, Bill, you're tops on that list. Laughing at stuff together was the first thing about you that made me swoon. It would not be the last. Thanks also to my sweet friend, Katie Green, who told me when Will was brand new, "You need to write this all down." Kids, you can blame Katie, because she's the one who planted the seed that I should write about you. It's *her* fault. I'm also thankful for parents who encouraged me and thought I could do anything. I have a book now to show for it, so that's not half bad. Thanks to my family for believing in me until I did.

I'd be remiss not to acknowledge my sweet children since every word written here was inspired by them. Willis and Lucy, when you turned my life on its head, I had no choice but to write about that. *A lot*. I hope you understand. And I hope you know that I love you more than all the words in this book—and all the thesauruses in the world—could ever say.

Don't be mad.

REFERENCES

Dedication quote page
1. Nora Ephron, *New Statesman and Society*, June 30, 1995, p. 32.
2. C. S. Lewis, quoted by Phillip Yancey, *What Good is God? In Search of a Faith that Matters* (New York: FaithWords, 2010), p. 100.

Part I: Trophies for Showing Up
1. Jill Churchill, *Grime and Punishment* (New York: Avon Books, 1989).

Part VII: Soapbox Rants and Neurotic Handwringing
1. Margaret Mitchell, *Gone with the Wind* (New York: Macmillan, 1936), p. 315.
2. Elizabeth Kolbert, "Spoiled Rotten," The *New Yorker*, July 2, 2012, http://www.newyorker.com/magazine/2012/07/02/spoiled-rotten.
3. Owen Gleiberman, Lisa Schwarzbaum, Chris Nashawaty, Kevin Sullivan, "16 Pixar Classics," *Entertainment Weekly*, August 8, 2013, http://www.ew.com/gallery/14-pixar-classics-we-rank-em/636287_3-toy-story-3-2010.

Part VIII: Lightning Bolts and Lightbulb Moments
1. A. A. Milne, *Winnie-the-Pooh* (New York: E.P. Dutton, 1926), p. 79.